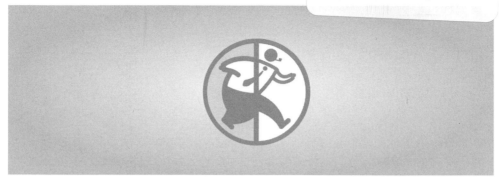

# Fat Daddy/Fit Daddy

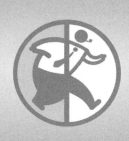

# Fat Daddy/Fit Daddy

## A Man's Guide to Balancing Fitness and Family

## Lawrence Schwartz

TAYLOR TRADE PUBLISHING
Lanham • New York • Toronto • Oxford

Published by Taylor Trade Publishing
An imprint of The Rowman & Littlefield Publishing Group, Inc.
4501 Forbes Boulevard, Suite 200
Lanham, Maryland 20706

Distributed by National Book Network

Library of Congress Cataloging-in-Publication Data

Schwartz, Lawrence, 1965-.
    Fat daddy, fit daddy : a man's guide to balancing fitness and family /
Lawrence Schwartz.— 1st Taylor Trade Pub. ed.
        p. cm.
    Includes index.
    ISBN 1-58979-039-1 (pbk. : alk. paper)
    1. Weight loss. 2. Physical fitness for men. 3. Fathers—Health and hygiene. I. Title.
RM222.2 .S358 2003
613.7'0449—dc21                                            2003012757

♾™ The paper used in this publication meets the minimum requirements of American National Standard for Information Sciences—Permanence of Paper for Printed Library Materials, ANSI/NISO Z39.48–1992.
Manufactured in the United States of America.

To my children, Cole and Cameron.

I love you.

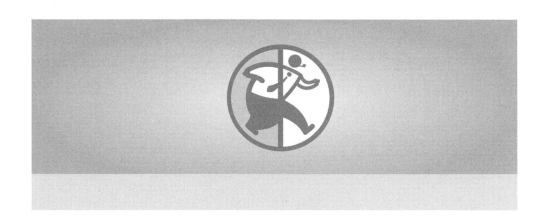

# Contents

## FOURTH QUARTER: HOW THE GAME IS WON

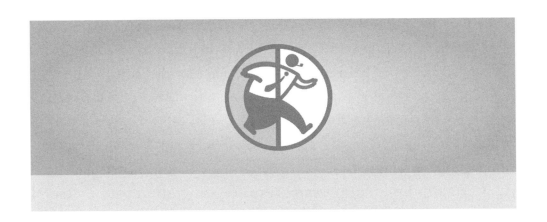

# Acknowledgments

Because *Fat Daddy* was written during the most difficult time in my life, I wanted first to acknowledge all of my dear friends and family whose unwavering love and support have helped me stay the course despite all the obstacles to completing this book. My best buddy Ray Balestri, who taught me to embrace discipline—and called me every week just to make sure I kept typing. My doctor friends Charles Wallace, M.D., and Jeff Whitman, M.D. (both dads). My brother Steve and his wife Julie, who's house became my Walden. And Patrick Brandt, who believed and supported me when all I was holding was a pair of twos in a game of five-card draw with jacks or better to open.

I would also like to thank all of the true professionals at Rowman & Littlefield Publishing Group for their steadfast support of *Fat Daddy*. From the publisher to the publicity department, to my editor extraordinaire Rick Rinehart—without all of your guidance, *Fat Daddy* would still be sitting on my hard drive. Thanks also to

Stacy Bratton and her amazing lens, to Arthur Eisenberg for his creative vision, and to Eric, Joe, and Tim for their careful reading, helpful suggestions, and humorous insights. Thanks also to Eisenberg & Associates for the logo and cover design, Salon Pompeo for styling for the cover photo, Jeff Crilley for public relations advice, Stacy Dail Bratton Photography for the cover photo, and Kent Winfield for website design and graphics.

Certainly, I must also express my deepest gratitude to my mom, who as a Holocaust survivor has shown me perseverance, and to my dad, who has always been my role model as a father. And last, but not least, I want to express my greatest love to my children Cole and Cameron, who in my darkest hours of doubt, showed to me all of what is good and pure in being a father.

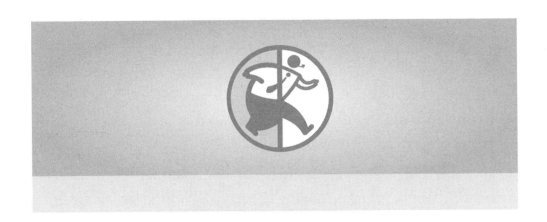

# Foreword

You might wonder why a plastic surgeon would write the foreword for a guide to fathers' fitness, diet, and family life. Actually, it's a natural fit. Plastic surgeons are the paint-and-body guys of medicine. We handle not only the well-publicized elective cosmetic procedures that make daily headlines but also the defects that result from all manner of injuries, cancers, infections, accidents, and years of neglect. This includes dealing with the results of men's remote-control, super-sized-meal lifestyles. In 2001, the last year for which statistics are available, surgical procedures for morbid obesity were up 48 percent over ten years ago. The number of male liposuction patients was up 29 percent over five years ago, and surgery for complications of diabetes (due to obesity)—food ulcers, amputations, and circulatory reconstruction—rose 40 percent from 1995. In short, I find myself operating on more and more Fat Daddies.

As a University of Texas graduate from the Earl Campbell era, I personally enjoyed reading Lawrence's *Fat Daddy*, and I could really relate to the sports analogies he used to illustrate his message. Being a Fat Daddy myself, I appreciate Lawrence's personal approach and found many simple, but overlooked, ideas and practical suggestions for managing one's circumference circumstances. This is a book that almost all of my male patients, friends, and, indeed, colleagues would do well to read and heed. There are plays in this book that every guy can incorporate into his own game plan.

The sports analogies Lawrence uses (and which I have adopted) will keep this message in the memory of nonliterary types and hold the interest of most people who need to hear the message in the first place.

But a further word on relevancy seems in order. In this book, Lawrence talks about man boobs. In my business it's not a joke at all. We refer to this particular phenomenon as *gynecomastia*. Unfortunately, because dads are fatter and fatter, gynecomastia is on the rise. In our Fat Daddy culture, about 35 percent of my liposuction patients are now men. And an unhealthy lifestyle can lead to far worse problems. I'm reminded of a recent example of an ex-jock CEO who simply didn't manage his diet; he may lose a foot due to uncontrolled gout and diabetes. This should call attention to the need for reading and heeding the Fat Daddy message.

Hopefully, *Fat Daddy* will be a "call to arms," as Manchester would say, at a time when post-dot-comers need it the most. Aside from the well-known problems of heart disease and cancer, there exists a plethora of less-well-publicized but nonetheless miserable maladies, such as premature arthritis, diabetes, and kidney disease, that can be at least partially overcome with planning, commitment, and execution of Lawrence's plan. *Fat Daddy*'s appeal to me, as a medical professional, is its encompassing approach to fitness, diet, and family.

In the sea of workout guides, relationship oracles, and diet diatribes, little, if anything, even makes an effort to tie it all together like *Fat Daddy* does.

My colleagues in plastic surgery and various other specialties love to quarrel over details of fitness plans. I can tell you, as a practicing physician who proffers advice daily to patients, family, and friends, Lawrence's advice is medically sound. Perhaps of equal importance, this book makes the package of solutions one we can actually implement—and live with.

Whether you believe in the low-fat, max-aerobic program, the Atkins' low-carb lifestyle, or any of the other numerous popular diet approaches, I personally encourage you to blend your chosen diet into Lawrence's meal-in-the-palm suggestion. This particularly applies to those of you who subscribe to the Atkins (or similar) low-carb, high-protein program. You will do better, short term and in the long haul, with smaller, sensible meals and fewer thirty-two-ounce porterhouse steaks. I strongly recommend that you commit to a personalized plan incorporating the *Fat Daddy* suggestions (preferably with the participation and approval of your personal physician) and, above all: do not quit! As a close friend's father observed of his aging friends (many of whom qualify as Fat Daddies and Fatter Granddaddies), quitting recreational sports and family involvement leaves only the quitting of breathing as a barricade to the next life.

As you implement the Fat Daddy proposition, I think it is encouraging to consider the numerous benefits of a plan that you and your family participate in. Most of us engaged in commercial enterprises are obsessed with the bottom line in our financial matters. The bottom line for Lawrence's game plan is simple: live longer, healthier, and happier. This means living to harass your kids as they face the Fat Daddy challenge themselves, having the strength to survive their teenage years, maintaining the love to share with your wife (or tolerate your ex), and managing the balance to keep it all in perspective. Finally, there is a great financial return. The fellow I mentioned earlier with the unattended gout and diabetes spent more than $1.3 million in one hospitalization trying to save his foot! With health care costs continuing to mount, taking personal responsibility and implementing a balanced plan have demonstrable economic benefits. No life is ever complete without the good physical and emotional health with which to enjoy all your other successes. Lawrence's sports analogy could be extended to say, "There is no next season."

A final word: There is uncommon wisdom in Lawrence's simple system, and his approach makes for an algorithm we can adapt to our own situations. Implement and improvise with your own favorite strategies, and, above all, make it fun—for yourself and for those around you. I really hope you enjoy reading *Fat Daddy* as much as I did.

CHARLES A. WALLACE, M.D.

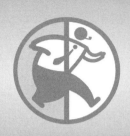

# FIRST QUARTER

# Game Plan

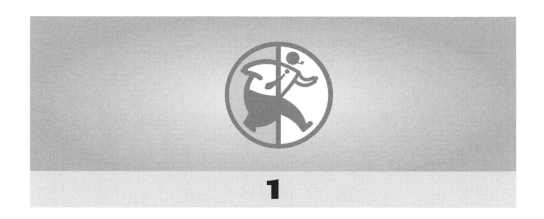

# Introduction

## It Happened

About a month after the birth of our first child, my wife and I went to the mall to shop for a new bathing suit. The swimwear was needed by yours truly. Forget all that claptrap Robert Bly wrote back in the early 1990s about how rugged men should sweat naked with each other in teepees but never, ever take their wives shopping for clothes. Trust me. Real men *do* ask their wives for fashion advice. So after nearly a year spent with my darling Mrs. Preggers—a wondrous year of nurturing her and sympathizing with her and learning about how utterly insane a pregnant woman can be—I felt it was time to return to my selfish man ways. Daddy wanted something new. Daddy needed his ego stroked. After a year of nesting, it was time to reintroduce the world to my abs of steel!

My wife pointed me in the direction of some "board shorts" that she'd seen the young bucks wearing on MTV. I picked out a pair in my usual size 32 and marched off to the dressing room. After tugging on the stretchy material, I strutted my way toward a three-way mirror where my stylist was waiting. I said, "What do you think?" She didn't need to answer. The look on her face said it all.

I thought at first that she might be suffering from some sort of *post*-postpartum depression. Maybe the color of the board shorts reminded her of the pillowcase in the delivery room. Who knows? Pregnancy and women confuse me.

Before I could ask her why she looked so disgusted, I turned and saw my reflection on the side panel of the mirror—and came face-to-face with my Great White Whale.

I can tell you now, years later and well into my recovery, that I had grown love handles. Contracted the Dunlap disease. Tied on a spare tire. Found my good partner Poncherello. But back then, standing in that department store, I couldn't believe it—a saddlebag! A big, honking, fat roll of man-stuffing cascading out of my swim-britches! I thought, "I'm only thirty-two. I'm still young and healthy. Still full of both vim and vigor. This can't be. The mirror is warped."

My wife tried not to stare, as if she was passing mangled wreckage on the highway. I couldn't blame her. I wanted to turn away, too. Even worse, though, I could see what lay ahead. The mirror acted like a magic window that looked into the future, I knew that this was just the appetizer to the inevitable daddy buffet. If drastic measures weren't taken, it would only be a matter of weeks before I had jowls, a waddle under my chin, tits so big I'd need a bra, and those freakishly pendulous earlobes that old men have.

I tried to ignore all this and refocus my wife's eyes on the board shorts. I sucked in my stomach. Did it help? Not much. The love handles were still there. I had to face reality; *we* had been eating for two.

Trying to ignore the belly of the beast, I mumbled, "I need to start doing some cardio work, huh?" "So you're getting a little soft," she said. "So what? You're a daddy now. It happens." Just like that, I knew "it" already had.

That was the truly depressing part. My wife—and most of my guy friends—saw this process as natural and unavoidable. I've found that most people believe the male progression is an unchangeable one: boys become men, who become husbands, who become Fat Daddies. I refused to buy into this myth.

That was a few years ago, and I must say my recovery has gone quite well and I was able to get my body back into some form of respectability. No, I don't have the 6-percent body fat that I had in my roaring twenties, but I now know how *not* to be a Fat Daddy.

I have documented my successes (and failures) in this book so other fathers can have a resource to turn to—when *it happens*.

Writing *Fat Daddy* was for me, in a real sense, self-therapy. After becoming a dad, I realized that fatherhood and fitness, unlike beer and pretzels, don't go together naturally. However, they can—and *should*. And as I've spoken with fellow Fat Daddies (most men over the age of thirty-five with munchkins), I've found that the easiest way to explain how fatherhood and fitness can be enjoyed simultaneously is to use a sports analogy (through my research, I have found that sports or sex are the easiest concepts for men to grasp; so for *Fat Daddy* we will use *sports* metaphors).

In *Fat Daddy*, we'll go with the analogy of the Big Game. I personally prefer to think the Big Game is played on the gridiron, because I'm short and stocky and don't exactly have what you'd call "mad hops." Here's how it works: Getting married, having kids, building a career, paying the mortgage, and trying to keep in shape are the plays. Love, happiness, and prosperity are how you keep score. However, it's the *staying in shape* part that can adversely affect the entire outcome of the game. To be truly mentally and physically fit, you need a game plan for success—and *Fat Daddy* is that plan. The plan is simple and it focuses on three essential elements—or *Keys to the Game*:

- **Food**—the foundation: composition, portion size, and frequency

- **Fitness**—the framework: time, place, and exercises

- **Family**—the fundamentals: exercising consistently as a family

Now don't get me wrong. I'll be the first to admit I don't have all the answers. But I do know that fatherhood is difficult and so is trying to stay in shape when you are pushing (or have passed) the age of thirty-five. There is never any time for yourself, and kids can be relentless. "Dad, are we there yet? Dad, I want a blue Power Ranger. Can we go to McDonalds? But I don't want to take a bath. I don't want to go to school today. Why can't I watch TV all day? Can I put my sister's head in the oven?" The questions and the demands go on and on (not to mention the soccer game that is conveniently scheduled on the Saturday that you need to go into the office and the babysitter canceled for later that night).

It's like playing defensive back and facing a running back who outweighs you by sixty pounds and keeps making the corner on your linebackers. So you've got to bring him down. And each time he runs you over and knocks your helmet sideways so you wind up looking through your ear hole. Then next play you've got to get up and go get run over by him again. With all of these demands on your time, with work and family, when is there any time for a dad to exercise?

Well, there is time, and it can be done. I know it can, not because I am a fitness expert, but because I'm a thirty-eight-year-old father of two who has figured out a smarter way to bring down that runner (hint: go for his legs). Just like you, I too have struggled to keep the waist measurement from far surpassing the inseam number on my Levi's while managing my career and other fatherly responsibilities (ladies wisely avoid this problem by simply assigning one number to the size of their jeans). However, making fitness a priority is a lifelong commitment, and it requires a great deal of patience.

Bottom line: I've broken down the wisdom of the diet and workout gurus and made an easy playbook for dads just like you and me to follow. That's it.

## So Where Did All These Fat Daddies Come From?

If you think about it, we men go through life pretty unprepared to meet the challenges that await us. Unprepared for that first punch in the nose on the blacktop, unprepared for our first orgasm, unprepared to handle the news that Lisa wants to be "just friends," unprepared for the responsibility (and drudgery) of our first "real" job, and *certainly* unprepared for fatherhood. Mainly we're not ready to be dads because from early on in our childhood society has told us not to ask for help, to figure it out on our own, because we're boys—and boys are *tough*.

But the reality is, boys grow up to become men who grow up to be dads (sometimes even Fat Daddies).

And there isn't just one type of Fat Dad.

There is the always-been-slightly-husky Fat Daddy, who, throughout his entire life, has always had what doctors refer to as a "lard ass." There is the ex-athlete Fat Daddy, who played running back for the bigger school across town and ran me over every single play and made me wish I was a cheerleader safe on the sideline and who never had an ounce of body fat until the one day he woke up with a paunch (and, I can only hope, knees as creaky and sore as mine). And, probably most common of all, there is the traveling Fat Daddy. This is also the most dangerous type of Fat Daddy because he picks up his bad habits while traveling on the road, trying to provide for his family. The traveling Fat Daddy eats comfort foods on an expense account, doesn't get enough sleep, and never has enough time to exercise. And there is no one around to keep tabs on what he's doing!

But regardless what type of Fat Daddy you are, as a father, you're a role model for your family (even if you're unprepared to play that role). Hey, if you spend most of your time plopped on the couch and watching TV, you can expect your clan to do the same. Study after study has shown that most Americans are out of shape or, worse, obese, and those bad habits are being passed along to the next generation. It's like a bad football team: poor front-office decisions, disinterested coaches, and bad practice habits lead to years, even decades, of disappointing results.

But it doesn't have to be this way, and *Fat Daddy* will show you how and why to do things differently.

From the first play, I want to tell you what this book is—and is not. As the subtitle emphasizes, *Fat Daddy* serves as a *guide* that describes a simple, no-nonsense approach to following a realistic eating plan, exercising for maximum gain while dedicating the minimum of time, while balancing family and work. That's it. The *Keys to the Game* are easy to understand, easy to follow, easy to remember, and will serve as a playbook to help busy dads cinch a couple of notches in that belt without a great deal of diet and workout sorcery. I guess you could say *Fat Daddy* is a condensed version of modern fitness principles that are geared for the complex realities of fatherhood.

## What Dads Will Learn

- The Reality Diet—how to eat normally, without counting carbs, points, or fat grams

- How better to fit in with your new teammates (mommy and baby)

- Exercise routines that can be performed in meetings, in the car, in a hotel room, on an airplane, and especially when you're with the kids

- Fitness routines that combine the easiest cardiovascular and strength principles

- Tips on budgeting time for exercise, prioritizing workouts, and managing stress

- Family fun fitness ideas

- Relaxation and yoga techniques that can be practiced anytime, anywhere

### How You'll Do It

After reading *Fat Daddy*, dads will learn how to:

- Make smarter food choices and learn about portion size

- Understand the different types of exercise regimens

- Find out how to dedicate more time in the day to exercise

- Exercise as a family

- Relax and better manage stress

## Calling Plays the Fat Daddy Way

I'm an average guy, from a middle-class family in Texas. I was not blessed with great abs, big calves, or broad shoulders. But, for the past twenty-five years (minus three when I was an out-of-shape fat dad), I have made fitness a priority in my life while I've stayed on top of my career *and* still managed to be an involved father (note: "involved" means more than just paying the bills). From my days as a jet-setting dot-com CEO ("Bubble? What bubble?") to being a soccer dad with my six-year-old, I have been able to maintain a fit, balanced lifestyle.  Maybe that's why the YMCA named me a Father of the Year in the Dallas area in 2003.

But it hasn't been easy. So, in 1998, I decided to write my first book, *The Professional's Guide to Fitness: Staying Fit While Staying on Track*, to help other busy professionals manage work and working out. The response was remarkable. Many busy professionals, men and women alike, wrote me to say that the book's simple concepts had helped them stay in shape while staying on track. So now five years have passed and I've decided to take what I've learned as a fitness enthusiast, a CEO, and a *father* to help other busy, overfed, stressed-out fathers get back in shape before they start having to pay for sex.

> "In January 2001, I weighed in at 242 pounds, about 60 pounds over my ideal weight. After getting a thorough physical, I decided to go on a sensible diet and start an exercise program. I also finally pulled your book out of the desk and read it. It was a great reinforcement for my journey. As you prescribed, I decided that I had to start "paying" myself rather than using the excuse that family and work were the only important things in life. Many of the topics outlined in your book hit really close to home. Thanks!"
>
> —DAN HUDSON,
> a dad from Dallas

## A Note about Format

As I sat down and outlined each chapter, I carefully selected what I think are the few essential fitness topics that I believe every father should know at least *something* about, and I left out everything else. Like advice on relationships. As you'll learn, I'm not USDA-certified in that area, so I'll leave that stuff to Dr. Phil (who, by the way, if I'm not mistaken, has put on a few lately). As I culled topics for *Fat Daddy*, I concentrated on information about **Food**, **Fitness**, and **Family** that men can put into practice in their everyday lives without having to seek outside assistance.

Essentially, since most guys are too busy and forget everything good for themselves, each topic in *Fat Daddy* is a bite-size chunk of useful information that dads can actually use. I liken them to Cliff's Notes on father-centric fitness concepts. And each chapter is designed, basically, so that it can be read during a morning bathroom event (if things have gotten so out of hand that you're not enjoying regular versions of the latter, then I'll leave that to Dr. Phil, too).

As I said, *Fat Daddy* uses the analogy that your life is like a football game. It's broken down into four quarters that build upon one another and are woven together by the *Keys to the Game*. Here's a look:

- **First Quarter**—the starting point: the "guy" mentality and why it's bad for our health

- **Second Quarter**—life changes: finding Mrs. Right, starting a family, and realizing you're a fat ass

- **Third Quarter**—the program: different workouts, diets, nutrition, and yoga

- **Fourth Quarter**—scoring points: tying the entire program together with your family

## The Keys to the Game: Food, Fitness, and Family

*Fat Daddy* explains in a simple, no-nonsense manner how to follow a realistic eating plan and do the minimum amount of exercise for maximum gains while balancing family and work. There are no calorie counters, no point systems, and no high-intensity workouts. The *Keys to the Game* are easy to understand, easy to follow, easy to remember, and are based on three areas: family (do it together and make it fun), fitness (schedule the time, find the proper place, and do some form of exercise), and food (when, how much, and what to eat).

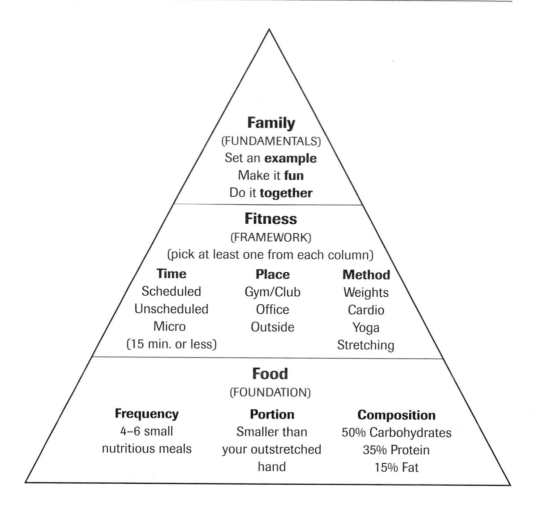

## Family—The Fundamentals

■ **Lead by Example.** As a father, it is your job to set the right example for your wife and children and to help them find the time and resources to get in shape *with* you. In *Fat Daddy*, dads will get tips on how to balance their most important asset—their family.

■ **Make It Fun.** As with everything else in life, having fun is the key to sticking with something. Even though Leisa Hart is nice to look at, exercising to the same *Buns of Steel* tape every morning, day in and day out, will get old quickly (though I must admit that I'm easily entertained and didn't get rid of my copy of *Buns of Steel 4* until I'd fairly well worn out the piece of carpet in front of our TV). But the best way to stay in shape is to vary your workout—every week head to the batting cages, play some golf (walk the course!), and maybe throw in a couple games of pickup basketball. *Fat Daddy* gives dads the road map for family fun workouts.

■ **Just Do It—*Together.*** It's a team game. If you work to help the entire family get or stay in shape, they will help you as well. Even if it's something as simple as setting fire to your Milky Way stash.

## Fitness—The Framework

■ **A Time and a Place.** Mornings at the gym, nights in your garage, lunch in your office. It doesn't matter where you exercise, so long as it doesn't get you arrested or fired. *Fat Daddy* suggests creative, time-friendly alternatives for squeezing exercise into a busy schedule. In *Fat Daddy*, busy dads will learn easy-to-follow routines that can be used in meetings, in the car, or even at the office.

■ **A Method to the Madness.** *Fat Daddy* shows busy dads how to break down exercise into *four* quarters, with *four* simple exercises per quarter, and how to find time to exercise *four* times per week—including the easiest and most important yoga poses, such as Downward-Facing Dog, Warrior, and the Plank.

## Food—The Foundation

■ **Frequent the Training Table.** Eat four to six small, somewhat healthy meals a day. Make it fun. Come up with names for your extra meals.

■ **Be Handy.** Here's another simple trick: Never eat more than your open hand at one sitting. Or, more precisely, never eat more than the *volume* of your open hand. For those daunted by spatial relations puzzles, if you're going to eat pizza, for example, that's about two slices.

■ **You Are What You Eat.** Watching what you eat can be a real pain, and it's not realistic for most dads. *Fat Daddy* reinforces simple, yet effective, nutrition tricks, like mnemonic devices to avoid bad habits ("if you eat after 8:00, you'll gain weight") and how to drink eight to ten glasses of water a day without drowning.

When you finish *Fat Daddy*, you will have learned fitness principles that are simple, practical, easy-to-follow, and most of all—effective. *Fat Daddy* will coach you along the way, helping you set realistic goals, teaching you "memory hooks" to be consistent with your daily routine, and training you to develop the determination to follow through. You will notice the positive changes not only in your physique but also in your overall quality of family and daily life.

So sit back (I mean sit up) and enjoy *Fat Daddy*. Do what you can. Try what you're comfortable with. Get your family involved. But stay with it.

Good luck. And remember: I'm on the sidelines, cheering you on!

---

### PLAYBOOK NOTES: Introduction

1. Becoming a Fat Daddy is normal, so relax.

2. Remember the *Keys to the Game*—Food, Fitness, and Family.

3. Read on.

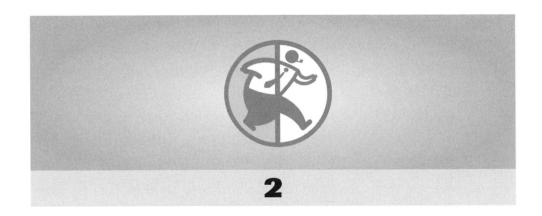

# 2

# The Original Game Plan

"Nobody in football should be called a genius. A genius is a guy like Norman Einstein."

> — JOE THEISMANN, former quarterback
> of the Washington Redskins and
> sports commentator for ESPN

In 1989, just out of college, I moved to Houston for my first "real job." I got my first apartment, about 600 square feet of bachelor-pad opulence, had total freedom, anything was possible, the world was my oyster, and I was utterly miserable. I was living in an unfamiliar city, and my college sweetheart had just left me because she said she needed space. (Stacy, I hope you found that space, and I hope it was cold and empty except for the scattered tiny bones of the other shrews who went there to die. Sorry. I got carried away.)

So there I was in Houston. I had about $300 in the bank, it was a couple days after Christmas, and I was all alone (cue soft music). I decided to do what any right-thinking, responsible guy would do:

I headed out for some cocktails. And not just a harmless night on the town to drown my sorrows but a bona fide, honest-to-goodness, certified bender that would hopefully include vomiting in my own shoes and waking up outdoors, naked.

I headed to a joint that was called, if memory serves, Club 6400. Real nice place. Great for throwing back some Bartles & James while nodding your head to Milli Vanilli (come on, girl, you know it's true). It was there, on that lonesome night, that I met my new best friend—literally. We'll call him Jeff, but on that night, he was Jefro (because in his drunken stupor he resembled a toothless hillbilly).

Well, while I was waiting in line to get into Club 6400, Jefro pushed his way ahead of me and said he was next. I should have kicked his ass, I know. Instead, though, probably due to my sorry emotional state, I let him cut in.

And, even odder, before we even got into the club, he started to sob on my shoulder and tell me *his* sad story about how *his* girlfriend had left him. And he offered me a beer from his coat pocket. Here was a guy, I thought, who had potential. We went inside and drank about our problems.

At some point in the evening, and after we'd sufficiently bonded but before I threw up, Jefro said, "You wanna go on a road trip?"

"Sure," I said. "When?"

"Tomorrow. Let's drive to Aspen for New Year's."

What the hell? I agreed.

Over the next few days, Jefro and I got to know each other pretty well. Thirty-six hours in a Honda Prelude and several cases of Budweiser will do that (author's note: don't try this with your wife). Space and decorum prevent me from sharing the details of that trip to Aspen, but the relevance for our purposes was that it was a part of the *Original Game Plan*.

The *Original Game Plan* is just that. It's the plan that most guys start out with—which happens to be *no plan*. We are spontaneous and prefer to take things as they come. Road trip! More shots! Suck the marrow out of life, and wait for the bones to fall in your lap. That same lack of planning applies to how we take care of our nutritional and fitness needs, too. We do what we want; eat what wanders by, workout when it's convenient.

Pizza for breakfast? No problem. Drive-thru burgers after a night of partying on the town with your buddies? No fat grams accumulated there. Snow bunny on the ski lift? Never regret that! It's all part of the *Original Game Plan*. Just hit the gym a couple hours more the next week and everything will balance out. Leave Aspen the next day, and you'll never have to talk to that girl again. In fact, John Gray, Ph.D., author of *Men Are from Mars, Women Are from Venus,* says men are hardwired to avoid making plans. And John Gray sold way more books than Robert Bly.

Our feelings—or lack thereof—govern our moods and habits and give us the ability to navigate the storms of life and our health and overall well-being (remember: we are unprepared for all of this stuff). So it's no wonder we don't have a clue that we are slowly training our lean, resilient bodies to turn into soft mounds of lint collectors. Put bluntly: "Men live sicker and die younger than women primarily due to diet." So says David Gremillion, M.D., director of the Men's Health Network.

What Dr. Gremillion's point illuminates is that as we get older, men's bodies require fewer calories. But most guys don't heed this type of advice, and their caloric intake stays the same or increases over time due to later dinners, more alcohol, and more vending machine comfort foods.

What this does *not* explain, but clearly suggests, is something that you already know intuitively: as men age, our metabolism slows down and we burn calories less efficiently. But since we have spent most of our lives as human garbage disposals, most of us keep on eating about the same amount, if not more.

And what's more, research has shown that the average man, father or not, puts on about 1 to 1.5 pounds every year. At that rate, a thirty-year-old stud will have grown a small child around his waist by the time he is fifty.

The bottom line—more calories without more exercise equals Fat Daddies.

But don't panic. Throughout *Fat Daddy*, you will learn simple techniques to shave a few extra calories out of your diet every day, while increasing the amount of calories you burn every day so you can keep that Buddha belly at bay. Yeah, you may gain some weight here and there over the next thirty years, but that is part of the *Original Game Plan*, too. It's called getting older.

When I was a high school footballer, our coach had a clever phrase that he hit us with during every halftime speech (along with every other high school coach in the country—sorry coach "Thompson"): "There is no 'I' in 'TEAM.'" My point is this: most sports require multiple guys wearing the same outfit. A team. And winning isn't about individuality or "I." However, in the *Original Game Plan*, for most guys, it's all about "I."

## The Playmaker

For most guys, the *Original Game Plan* also includes a fierce desire for upward mobility in their careers. Guys graduate college, get that first job, and work like hell—fifty-, sixty-, or even eighty-hour weeks. First in, last out, lunch at the desk, press the shirt for another day.

And why do we bust our humps and put in the hours at the sawmill? "Rovers Law": because we can (don't worry, you'll get it in a minute) and we want to be successful. At this point in our lives, we really have no motivation to please anyone except ourselves (did

I hear an oink?). We work our asses off because we are young, full of spit and vinegar, and we want to climb the corporate ladder all the way to the corner office.

But hard labor, endless work hours, and the obsessive pursuit of our career goals can turn a man into a workaholic, and that ain't good (I know, because I've been one). Self-confessed workaholics speak of using work as a way to cope with life, just as alcoholics use alcohol. And if you have any of the symptoms below, you should seek a good therapist:

- You work nights, weekends, and always bring work home with you

- You feel guilty when you are not working

- Your list of priorities does not include relaxation

- You forget anniversaries, birthdays, and other important events

- You accept more work even though you are overcommitted

- You work to escape problems

- You are always tethered to a pager, cell phone, or Blackberry

- You have few friends or hobbies outside of work

One of my friends likened the *Original Game Plan* to the Death Star from *Star Wars*, using its tractor beam to pull us toward selfishness, bad eating habits, just-in-time workout programs, and obsessive work habits. We just can't stop it.

And, speaking of friends, don't think your friends can offer you solace. Your friends (and the process of parting with them) are part of the *Original Game Plan*, too.

## Original Teammates

Remember when you had lots of friends? Guy friends, girl "friends," friends at work, family friends, and beer-drinking friends. Different friends to help you enjoy and validate your own pursuit of hedonism. Being a friend meant a lot. It meant rehashing together an amazing play at the ballpark or an amazing play on a date the night before. I recently saw Bill Cosby in concert, and he said his wife complained that he was a hermit and didn't have any friends. He replied, "Hell, I did, but you ran them all off." I can see Cosby's point, because in the *Original Game Plan*, guys have many friends. But as guys become men, and men become dads, your true friends turn out to be your family and a small group of confidants that you can count on one hand. And since that trip to Aspen, Jeff still has my thumb (does that sound dirty?).

## Fourth and Long

So let's summarize: In the formative years of defining who we are and making a name for ourselves, guys are dogs—plain and simple. We are (were) pretty unprepared for everything that is thrown our way, we are selfish, we have no regard for diet, and we treat our bodies like crap most of the time (but, unlike dogs, try as we might, we can't lick ourselves). We become workaholics and gluttons for every crappy experience life can throw our way. But through determination, intimidation, intuition, skill, or luck, we find our way. All to one day share with a fair maiden in a white dress to start a family with. And that, too, is part of the *Original Game Plan*. However, the *Original Game Plan* doesn't work forever, and to be successful in the next part of the game you will have to punt your old habits.

## PLAYBOOK NOTES: The Original Game Plan

1. The *Original Game Plan* is for guys only—no daddies allowed.

2. You have to start taking stock of your diet and the amount of exercise you get before it's too late.

3. Too much work can kill you, so pace yourself.

4. When you find Mrs. Right you will have to punt the *Original Game Plan.*

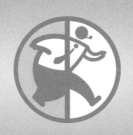

# SECOND QUARTER

# Change in Strategy

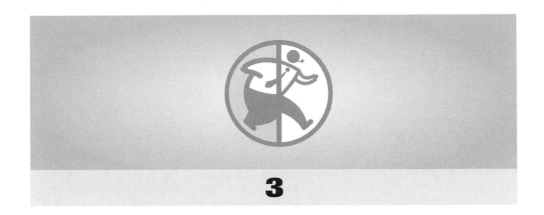

# 3

# The New Game Plan

"When in doubt, punt!"
—JOHN HEISMAN

## Changing Plays

One morning, you will wake up to a whole new ball game. Here's how you'll know when things have changed: A girl will be lying next to you in bed, and not only will you remember her name, but, even more surprising, you won't immediately want to kick her out of your house. On the contrary, you'll find yourself watching this wonderful creature as she sleeps, hoping that when she wakes up the two of you can just spend all Sunday morning sitting around in your underwear, reading the paper, talking about which matinee you should catch. You'll know that she takes her coffee with a lot of milk but only a little sugar and a dollop of whipped cream. This is when you know you're in trouble, and the *Original Game Plan* won't work.

The *Original Game Plan*, remember, was designed to handle all-night poker parties with the guys. The *Original Game Plan* worked great when it came to convincing that chick in New Orleans to let you take her pants off in the Port-A-Pottie at Jazz Fest. The *Original Game Plan* was driving in reverse in the drive-thru line at midnight and committing class-A misdemeanors and calling around to bars the next day to find your credit card.

The *Original Game Plan* has no contingency for the woman lying in bed next to you, whom, your tingling Spidey Sense suggests, you—gulp—love. It's time to install a whole new offense, my friend. The *New Game Plan* is about understanding that your value system is changing. It's about settling down with a life partner. The *New Game Plan* brings consistency where once there was chaos, companionship where there was solitude, and commitment rather than awkward sex in a portable bathroom with a castoff from a *Girls Gone Wild* video.

In other words, we're talking maturity (here is where I'm thankful my parents don't get space for rebuttal—but just bear in mind that Tom Landry didn't need to be able to throw a sixty-yard TD pass to be a good coach).

The *New Game Plan* brings into play the *real* Keys to the Game, starting with Food, Fitness, and Family. For simplicity's sake, throughout the book, I will break the Keys to the Game down first by topic (such as Food, Fitness, and Family), and then by different observations, strategies, and tactics within those topics.

### The Fundamentals—Family

Finding a life partner is not a simple task. Every man wants his wife to have a sense of humor, a warm personality, an inquisitive mind, and strong family values. On top of all that, it would be nice if she had a really choice set of chest hams. The point is, though, as difficult as scouting your new teammate is, that just might be the easy part. Staying together is the tough part. I ain't the only one having trouble doing it. In our country, more than 50 percent of all marriages end in divorce (according to the National Center for Health Statistics). In Europe, the failure rate is less than half of that (probably because of the mandatory three-year waiting period).

Anyway, just as in every game that is played on a field, court, rink, or squared circle, you learn more in the game of love when you lose. At least I hope I've learned a few things.

However, researchers believe some of the most common synergistic qualities that have kept couples together the longest have been:

■ Mutual respect and kindness

■ Similar faith

■ The ability to be a good listener

■ Similar family upbringing

■ Sweating the small stuff (trying to make the other person happy—little things matter)

And, finally, if you still don't think I know what I'm talking about, I'd like to point out that I'm related to Sigmund Freud (my mother's grandfather's first cousin, no kidding). And even the great Sigmund Freud even confessed a deep frustration with the opposite sex: "The great question, which I have not been able to answer despite my thirty years of research into the feminine soul, is, what does a woman want?"

## The Framework—Fitness

On to the stuff that's easier to get a handle on. If the family is the basic fundamentals of a healthy dad, then fitness is the framework.

If your *Original Game Plan* consisted of a couple weekly trips to the gym, then you're not in trouble—but the "Check Engine" light is on. The new guidelines commissioned by the Institute of Medicine, a prestigious organization that advises the government on medical matters, says everyone should have at least an hour of moderately intense physical activity each day—twice the amount of exercise the U.S. surgeon general called for in 1996 (*Dallas Morning News*, September 6, 2002, pg. 1-A). Pretty shocking, huh?

But as Dr. Benjamin Caballero, of Johns Hopkins University, pointed out, "The one hour can be split throughout the day and can include ordinary activities" (*Dallas Morning News*, September 6, 2002, pg. 1-A). We'll delve a lot deeper into different types of exercises, body types, and how to squeeze in more time for fitness later in the book, but for now here are the basics of the *New Game Plan*.

The general notion of fitness can be broken down into three areas: *strength*, *endurance*, and *flexibility*. *Strength* is the amount of force that a muscle group can exert in a one-time burst of effort (like weight lifting); *endurance* is the ability to overcome fatigue and to exercise over a period of time (like jogging or swimming); and *flexibility* is how well your muscles and joints move through a full range of motion. It's the goal of *Fat Daddy* simply to explain to overworked, overstressed, and overfed dads how to improve in these three areas of fitness, with proper nutrition and quality family activities.

### The Foundation—Food

Let's face it. Most guys (dads included) eat like crap. But it's never too late to change your diet and start eating more healthy foods. For the purpose of this chapter, I will touch on the basics. We'll go into more detail about food choices, fad diets, and the Reality Diet in the Third Quarter, *The Training Table*.

The *Fat Daddy* eating plan is extremely easy to follow and has no special meals to buy and no points to count. It's based entirely on:

- **Portion size** (how much)

- **Meal frequency** (how often)

- **Food composition** (what)

And why is food so important? I like to refer to food (or nutrition) as the "foundation" of the *Keys to the Game*. But first let's start off with a frame of reference.

Study after study has shown that most Americans are out of shape or, worse, obese, and they pass their bad habits along to the next generation. It's like the Cincinnati Bengals. They're losers. And even new players who have talent pick up that loser mentality when they're drafted. (Hopefully, Carson Palmer will change all that.)

Those new players, of course, are our kids. That's where bad habits create real trouble. A recent survey by the National Association for Sport and Physical Education found that only 44 percent of children participate in school-based physical activity on a daily basis, and 5 percent receive no physical education at all. What's more, the percentage of children between six and eleven who are overweight has more than doubled since 1970, according to the most recent figures from the National Center for Chronic Disease Prevention and Health Promotion. Can you say "juvenile diabetes"? So, the *New Game Plan* is designed not just to get you healthy and happy but to teach your kids how to play right, too.

## Portion Size

There has been much debate about calorie consumption, food combining, and the like. Forget all that. The *Fat Daddy* rule of thumb says: If the amount of food on your plate is greater than the size of your hand, then your portion is too big (more on this later).

### Frequency

Think of your stomach as a furnace. The more fuel you add to the fire, the hotter it will burn and the more fuel it will consume. When you eat small, nutritious, frequent meals throughout the day, you are adding fuel to the fire. Your body says, "Hey, food is coming in so fast that I should speed up the metabolism to prepare for the next feeding." So what happens? Your body begins metabolizing food at a faster rate, instead of storing fat to prepare for starvation.

Eating small, more frequent meals will also help your body regulate blood sugars, which will create a more consistent energy level. Throughout *Fat Daddy*, you will learn how to eat more (four to six) smaller nutritious meals a day and actually lose weight!

### Composition

New research by the Institute of Medicine has determined that the healthiest diets should get about half their calories from carbohydrates, one-quarter to one-third from protein, and the rest from fat. Remember it this way: If you can pick it, pluck it, peel it, or hook it, you're probably okay. Proper food choices are one of the most essential *Keys to the Game*.

Not only is focusing on portion, frequency, and composition far simpler than trying to follow a fad diet, but it works better over the long run. Feel free to try to "Eat All You Want and Still Lose Weight!" or "Melt Fat Away While You Sleep!" The weight-loss industry in America generates $33 billion in all manner of pills, potions, gadgets, and programs that hold the promise of a slimmer, happier future. You're welcome to contribute to that industry. But studies show that while men who try fad diets may shed a few of their *Original Game Plan* pounds, very few—perhaps 5 percent—will manage to keep all of it off in the long run (and this only gets worse as time rolls on).

## Why Dieting Is a Trick Play That Never Works

Diets restrict eating solely to lose pounds. Eating less slows down your metabolism. Basically it prepares your body for starvation. Your body starts to use all foods as an energy reserve and stores them as fat. You're eating less and you're losing weight, but your body has begun to operate differently. So once you stop the diet and start eating normally again, the body says, "Hey, fat cells, eat up! We need to prepare for the next starvation period (diet)." It's like pouring water on a dry sponge; the body's fat cells swell and prepare for the worst. The body also retains water that your desperate carbohydrate cells were deprived of when you cut calories. You wind up feeling bloated and like you're about to have your period (yah, I know, *gross*). That's why they call it a "diet"—you DIE ON IT.

The bottom line is that the *New Game Plan* will require some changes. Changes in the way you eat, how you behave. But the *New Game Plan* is really a pretty easy offense to learn. It's about growing up, realizing you need to take better care of yourself, and finding your life partner.

"I was just getting out of grad school when I met my wife. She was a teacher and so she was off for the summer. I was still working a part-time job as a bartender on weekends. We had lots of free time, and one thing we would do as a date was to go to a health club where we both belonged to and work out. We'd follow that up with a couple of drinks at the bar next door for happy hour and who knows what for later. Back then, life was pretty easy."

—DENIS POMBRIANT. a dad from Boston

However, once you find Mrs. Right and you make munchkins together, the challenges get tougher—so you'd best study the *Keys to the Game* now!

## PLAYBOOK NOTES: The New Game Plan

1. Understand the *Keys to the Game:* **Food, Fitness,** and **Family**.

2. **Food** is the foundation and is based upon portion size, meal frequency, and meal composition.

3. **Fitness** is the framework and is comprised of strength, endurance, and flexibility.

4. Having a healthy **Family** is fundamental to good health and well-being.

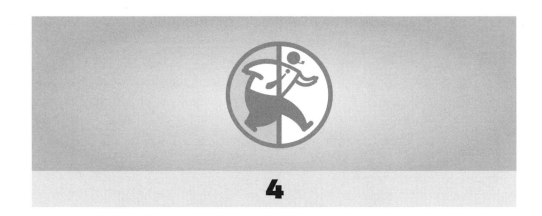

# 4

# Your New Teammates

"People who work together will win, whether it be against complex football defenses or the problems of modern society."
—VINCE LOMBARDI, former head football coach of the Green Bay Packers

Where do I start? The day I got married? Or the day I became a father? Both were major draft picks that dramatically changed my life and my midriff.

The classics are filled with romantic stories about couples who were meant for each other, who fell in love at first sight, under charmed circumstances. Take *Animal House*, for instance. When Mayor DePasto's daughter busts Pinto for trying to shoplift sundry cuts of meat from a grocery store, and when he invites her to the party at the Delta House that night, you know the two were meant for each other. Never mind that they wound up making the sign of the two-backed beast on the fifty-yard line of Faber's football field. And so what if she was only thirteen? You got the impression that their al fresco union meant something and that Pinto would wait for her—at least until she got her license.

## Mrs. Right?

The story of how I met my wife wasn't quite as romantic. I was twenty-six years old and cruising a bar in Dallas with my older brother Steve. And there I saw her—Mrs. Right. Her hair was long and golden brown, her smile was bright as a beacon, and her eyes twinkled like stars on a clear Texas night. Plus she was an easy mark because she'd had a lot to drink. Our first conversation, in fact, was about beer. She said something about how the beer I was drinking had 300 calories in it. I used to work for a beer company and knew she was wrong. I let her argue her point for a while, then simply showed her the label. Charming, huh?

Seriously, though, I remember telling my brother that he'd better back off. I knew right then that I'd met my wife. Amy was fun-loving and had a warm heart. It's hard to explain and sounds like a cliché, but my heart went up into my throat, and I really did fall in love at first sight. Right then, The *New Game Plan* went into full effect.

Now, of course, I'm no longer twenty-six and I'm no longer married. Love at first sight is a wonderful thing, but the years have taught me that it doesn't guarantee you'll grow old and happy together. As human beings, we are not really wired for long-term commitments. Courtship is natural. Sex is natural. Intimacy is natural. Long-term togetherness is not. Which isn't to say that it's not something worth striving for (how's that for a ringing endorsement?).

One reason that staying together can be worth the effort: Mrs. Right may actually be good for your health. Research has shown tremendous health benefits for guys who tie the knot. Not only in physical and mental health but in longevity as well. Jessie Bernard wrote in *The Future of Marriage*, "there is improved mortality and health rates for married men compared to unmarried men, and higher reported levels of happiness and mental wellbeing for married men compared with both unmarried men and married women." More precisely, divorced, single, and widowed men live significantly shorter lives than married men. Why? No research has really pinpointed the reason, but eating a more consistent diet (of healthier, home-cooked meals), more exercise, less stress, and more sex are all likely factors.

But after the wedding bells stop clanging and you and your Mrs. Right settle into your comfort zone, the pitfalls to fitness start. Since they are off the market, most married men tend to lose the eye of the tiger (cue *Survivor* and enter Rocky, in gray sweats jogging). They want to relax and spend more time on the couch than in the gym.

And this, brothers, is the first major fumble.

Just as in sports, when you start to get comfortable, you get sloppy. When it looks like you're winning the game, you slack off a little, you don't try quite as hard, and your defense soon becomes your offense. And you know what? That's when injuries happen. And the snatching of defeat out of the jaws of victory becomes almost inevitable.

But, as you will learn in the *Keys to the Game*, it doesn't have to be that way. Rather than have Mrs. Right contribute to your demise, you can make her a participant in a healthy lifestyle. It will take some time and practice. Sure. We'll touch on family workouts and better nutritional habits later in the book, but for now:

- **Make time for exercise.** Earlier in the morning or later in the evening—it doesn't matter. Just get at least one hour of exercise at least six days a week.

- **Do it together.** Couples that work out together stay together.

- **Eat dinner early.** If you eat after 8:00 P.M., you will gain weight (and if the glove fits, you must acquit). Plus, having a consistent time for dinner together is great for communicating and bonding.

## Your #1 Draft Pick

When my Mrs. Right told me that we were pregnant with our first child, I was the happiest I've ever been. I remember it vividly. It was the winter of 1996, and we were in the Whitehall Hotel in Chicago (great digs, by the way). I guess you could say I had that typical reaction that most guys get when someone tells them for the first time that they are going to be a father: "OH SHIT!"

My knees buckled, I felt flush, and my whole childhood raced up and ran over me right there—my childhood was officially behind me—I had crossed over to being a dad. Additionally, to show Amy exactly how happy I was, I lost control of my bowels.

I was going to be a father—of a boy! Now *that* did make me happy. What an incredible sigh of relief. I did it! I propagated my family name. But would he have dark hair like his daddy or blond hair like his mommy? (He ended up having red hair like his grandpa.) Would he become an athlete someday? A fireman or doctor or maybe even president? (This was before the Starr Report, remember.)

As a young father, all of these things and more go through your head—and it can be overwhelming. There is actually a name for this confusing period when a man first discovers he's going to be a dad. It's called *couvade* (pronounced coo-vahd). Couvade is a developmental stage for men that, in some cases, can lead to guys having depression, sympathy pains, taking to bed rest, and even gaining weight. And, speaking of weight, it sneaks up on you—fast!

## The Sneak

Early on, even before Mrs. Right and I were married and decided to have children, we both agreed that we'd each equally participate in the pregnancy, the labor, the birth, and the raising of the children.

I drew the line at having an episiotomy, but we did go to Lamaze class, decorated the nursery, and did the whole baby shower thing together. I was into it. Really, *too* into it. When Mrs. Right got pregnant, she went from being an athletic 5-foot-6, 115-pound gazelle to being a rotund 175-pound—let me choose my animal comparison carefully here, lest it come back to haunt me—water buffalo. This woman liked to eat! And with all of that food around, it was only a matter of time before some of it started to *sneak* my way.

It wasn't so much the nutritious breakfast that we had every morning (nutrition is key for a growing baby) or the hearty dinner we shared every night. It was the stuff that sneaked through the cracks (go easy, you fans of the dirty double entendre). It was all of the new extra "craving food" we had around the house. It was the Twinkies, the chocolate, the ice cream, all of the multiflavored juices, the pizza for appetizers. And I don't want to leave out a

> **KEY PLAY**
>
> The American College of Obstetricians and Gynecologists say that moderate exercise is good during pregnancy if approved by a doctor.

dozen powdered donuts every other day. Even though she worked out, Mrs. Right was an eating machine. Sticking with the *Animal House* theme, think Blutarsky going through the line in the lunchroom, before he turns himself into a human zit.

And what was I supposed to do? Just stand there and watch her? I nibbled a little here and a little there, and the next thing I knew— well, you remember the dressing room with the swim trunks incident. Mrs. Right lost her "baby weight," but I didn't.

## Eating for Two

Your wife probably knows all of these things already, but aside from all the pickles and ice cream, there are very important guidelines to follow when your wife has a bun in the oven. During your wife's pregnancy, she will need a lot for energy. Overall, it may take up to 80,000 calories to make a baby! What's more, there are some very specific nutrients she will need as deemed appropriate by the Institute of Medicine, National Academy of Sciences:

- **Protein.** She will need about 10 extra grams of protein each day. A roast beef or turkey sandwich should do the trick.

- **Fat.** Although fats need to be watched closely, they are an important energy source. They also will help Junior's brain and eye development.

- **Carbs.** Carbohydrates, like whole grains and plant foods, will supply the baby with a variety of essential vitamins and minerals and will be a good source of fiber for mom (oh, smell the joy!).

- **Iron.** Iron helps carry oxygen to cells and tissues and aids in making new red blood cells. And, since blood volume increases by approximately 50 percent during pregnancy, iron becomes critical. Some plant foods have good sources of iron, but your best bet is a juicy steak.

- **Folic Acid.** No, this is not a new designer party drug. Folic acid is critical for the body to make new cells, especially the neural tube (this is what turns into the spinal cord). Foods like citrus fruits and juices, dark green leafy vegetables like spinach, and enriched grains like bran cereal are all very high in folic acid.

- **Calcium.** Just like adults, babies need calcium for strong teeth and bones. Also, your wife's skeletal structure will be supporting extra weight and will need to be reinforced during her pregnancy. Calcium helps with both. Most dairy products are very good sources of calcium.

■ **B Vitamins.** B vitamins are essential to unleash energy in the foods you eat. Most lean beef, pork, and poultry are good sources of B vitamins.

**KEY PLAY**

When it comes to anything that has to do with pregnancy, always consult a physician first.

■ **Vitamin C.** Studies have shown that getting enough vitamin C during pregnancy may reduce the risk of pregnancy-induced hypertension and miscarriage. Again, citrus fruits and juices and even peppers (red, green, or yellow) are good sources of vitamin C.

■ **Prenatal Vitamins.** These should be one of the first things that your doctor mentions.

Below is a table of most of the critical nutrients your Mrs. Right will need during pregnancy as determined by the Food and Nutrition Board at the Institute of Medicine, National Academy of Sciences in 2001.

|  | NORMAL | PREGNANT |
|---|---|---|
| Calories | 2200 | 2500 |
| Protein (g) | 45-60 | 60 |
| Iron (mg) | 18 | 27 |
| Folate (mcg) | 400 | 600 |
| Calcium (mg) | 1000 | 1000 |
| Zinc (mg) | 8 | 11 |
| Choline (mg) | 425 | 450 |
| Niacin (mg) | 14 | 18 |
| Riboflavin (mg) | 1.1 | 1.4 |
| Thiamin (mg) | 1.1 | 1.4 |
| $B_6$ (mg) | 1.3 | 1.9 |
| $B_{12}$ (mcg) | 2.4 | 2.6 |
| Vitamin C (mg) | 75 | 85 |

# Becoming Second String

Many people have said that once there are children in the mix, dads end up riding the pine. Not only do we become second string, but we get penalized with diaper duty, puke on our tie, and sleep deprivation—akin to some of the same tactics the National Security Agency uses when interrogating suspected terrorists. It's bad. And there is no manual, website, book, or friend that can really prepare you for the first months with a newborn.

Oh, and don't forget the worst part about being second string: Mrs. Right's breasts will grow to such size that Goodyear could put a pilot in them and fly them over sporting events. But you can't touch 'em. Nope. There all for Junior. He's first string.

But, on the bright side, we dads are now living in a mom's world. And once a woman becomes a mom, the transition of power is swift and decisive. So in a sense, most of the time we are rescued (or reassigned) from our daddy duties because we appear not to be "getting it right." Herein lies a great opportunity. While Mrs. Right is being mom, you can slowly get yourself (and your new teammates) interested in fitness again.

And here's how to start off nice and easy:

- **Get the mound moving.** While your Mrs. Right is pregnant, being physically active will help improve her circulation, may prevent those nasty varicose veins, and should help prevent excess weight gain—not to mention give her more energy.

- **Lead by example.** Start the team moving again and getting back to a normal routine. Healthy, happy parents are one of the greatest gifts to give your kids (regardless of whether you are married or not).

■ **Toss it.** Toss out the remaining junk food and shop with your spouse for groceries. You can make healthier choices together.

■ **Play a lot.** Nothing is better than fun for dissipating tension and forging trust and good relationships with babies and your spouse.

■ **Take advantage of your baby's portability.** Don't be afraid to pick up your baby—a lot. Aside from the bonding benefits, he or she probably weighs eight to twelve pounds.

■ **Get out.** Stimulation is good for kids, and babies make great adventure companions. Besides, you'll get lots of attention from women who would have never acknowledged you before.

Just remember, the longer you wait to get back in shape, the harder it's going to be. So don't ignore the warning signs. If it's painful to look at yourself in the mirror with your shirt off, then it's time to make some changes. If you've let things go to the point that you can't see the instrument you used to get your wife pregnant, then for God's sake, do something before the coach calls you into his office and tells you that you won't be making the trip to Sunday's game. Know what I'm saying?

> "Having a baby transports the parents into a kind of endless hour-after-hour journey that ultimately lasts two or three years. At least for me, the absence of sleep triggered a need for high-calorie meals and snacking. There is a feeling of having the right to eat lots of forbidden foods. You are working so hard. There is nothing as scrumptious as a hearty breakfast of fried eggs and bacon after a late night feeding, midnight bottle, and 5:00 A.M. diaper change!"
>
> —TONY ADAMS,
> a dad from Connecticut

## PLAYBOOK NOTES: Your New Teammates

1. When you find Mrs. Right, you'll know it.

2. Mrs. Right will be the player who will actually deliver the #1 draft pick—so treat her with love and respect.

3. Watch out for the sneak—foods that mysteriously find their way to you.

4. When you have your #1 draft pick, you become second string—so get used to it.

5. Lead by example and help get you and your spouse back on the fitness track.

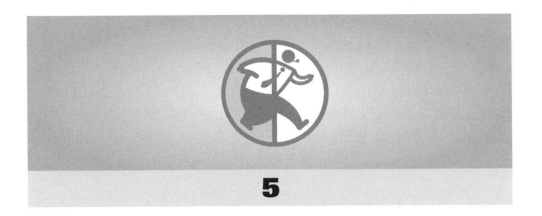

**5**

# Penalty! Illegal Love Handles, Saddlebags, and Man Boobs

"If there is going to be a fat guy around here it's going to be me."

— BILL PARCELLS, Dallas Cowboys head coach,
during his first off-season with the team

## This Is Not My Equipment

When a guy gets a flag for having turned into a Fat Daddy, he does what every great athlete does: He argues the call. He gets in the ref's face and, using language that would shock a trucker, he tells him just how bad the call is. Then, after he's worn himself out complaining, he concedes and takes the penalty and confidently says he can get back in shape if he wants to. "It's only a couple of pounds, no big deal." I know, because that's what happened to me when I was trying to outfit myself with the swim britches.

Fine. Get it out of your system. Then face reality. If you stand shirtless in front of a mirror and see breasts staring back at you, you can either shave them and try to get work as a bra model, or you can face the fact that you have officially turned into a Fat Daddy. The decision is yours. Also keep in mind, though, that man boobs aren't the only signs of a Fat Daddy. Belt-busting beer bellies and love handles are actually the most frequent evidence of our unhealthy habits.

## The Scouting Report

Fat Daddies are not born; they are made—over time. And, unfortunately in the United States, we're making more and more of them. New research by the *Journal of the American Medical Association* found that greater than 30.5 percent of Americans are obese, up from 22.9 percent a decade ago. Nearly two-thirds fall short of obese but qualify as overweight. Of those, almost half are men. And a recent Framingham Heart Study found that a man carrying just twenty-two extra pounds has a 75 percent greater chance of having a heart attack than a guy at his ideal weight. Just gaining eleven to eighteen pounds can double the risk of developing type 2 diabetes.

On the bright side, a study by the Cooper Clinic for Aerobic Research in Dallas found that unfit men who increased their fitness over a five-year period lowered their mortality rate by 44 percent compared with those who did nothing. That figure alone should make every "fitness challenged" dad get off his ass and try to get in better shape.

## Body Types: Running Backs, Linemen, and Kickers

Now before you sink too far into a pit of despair and go get a gallon of tin roof ice cream to eat while you watch *Fried Green Tomatoes*, you need to understand how different body types change as they grow older. Basically, everyone starts life as one of three body types, or somatotypes. Somatotypes play a significant role in how we put on fat and build muscle. Knowing which group you belong to will help you set goals and manage your own expectations.

**Mesomorphs** are running backs. They are usually very muscular and defined. They have broad shoulders, small waists (damn I'm jealous), and thick joints. Think Eddie George or Jevon Kearse. Mesomorphs face weight gain in the later stages in life—surprise. Most of this gain can be attributed to poor nutrition and lack of activity. They run into trouble later in life because most mesos, when they're young, get used to staying in shape with little effort. But then their bad habits catch up to them, and mesos become the Ex-Athlete Fat Daddy.

**Endomorphs** are lineman. Here we're talking about the Always Been Fat Fat Daddy. Most endos tend to have thin limbs and a round middle. However, their smaller limbs can give them great speed and agility. That's why many NFL linemen actually have relatively small legs compared with the rest of their bodies. Unfortunately, because of their slower metabolism, endomorphs have a greater propensity to pack on pounds and spend their entire life working or dieting to control their weight.

**Ectomorphs** are kickers. They eat all they want, drink all they want, and they still stay skinny (mainly because they have fast metabolisms). Those lucky bastards. All I can say to my endo and meso brothers is that you've got to get yourself on the kickoff return team and hit those sissies hard enough to make them go back to playing soccer. Ectos do have other disadvantages too. Besides looking like a coat hanger, they're more prone to injuries, and they sometimes lack energy.  Some famous ectomorphs might resemble Randy Moss or Jerry Rice (or if you need a better visual, how about Elle McPherson or Heidi Klum). But, all things considered, an ecto has the best opportunity to sculpt a lean muscular physique and stay leaner longer.

## Busted Plays

As I said, Fat Daddies aren't born; they're made. And, usually, they're made from one of the following three busted plays (any combination of two or more of these factors will guarantee that you'll become a Fat Daddy):

**Busted Play #1:** Bad Diet + Lack of Exercise  = **Fat Daddy**

**Busted Play #2:** Pregnant Wife + More Food  = **Fat Daddy**

**Busted Play #3:** Job + Responsibility + Stress = **Fat Daddy**

Turn your attention to the Telestrator, if you will, and let's break down these busted plays.

### Busted Play #1

What exactly is a bad diet, and how much exercise do we really need? We'll dissect all of the different diets and workout routines in the third quarter, but for now let's concentrate on the basics.

*Stick with Smaller Portions.* Forget all those fad diets that severely restrict the number of calories or types of food you can consume. Studies have shown that they are ineffective in the long term. Not only will you gain back the weight you lost, but you'll probably pack on a few more pounds in the process.

When trying to lose or maintain your weight, you can eat pretty much anything—so long as you practice portion control and you exercise regularly. In fact, it is important to enjoy a variety of foods. When you eliminate certain types of food completely, they become more tempting, which may push you to binge on them, given the opportunity. Put a plate of pasta in front of someone who's been eating nothing but meat and cheese for two months. See what happens.

Eating reasonable amounts of food in a super-sized biggie world can be difficult. Here are some tips to help you control your portions when you eat at home and when you dine out.

1. **Hand job.** Use your outstretched hand as a visual aid to determine an adequate portion of food on your plate. If you can't cover it with your hand, don't eat it.

2. **Make one trip.** In order to simplify this task, don't put an over-abundance of food on the table. If the recipe serves four but only two people are eating, store the extra portions immediately. In particular, avoid putting too many plates with different types of food on the table. If you dig into a bunch of different foods ("European style"), you're much less likely to be aware of how much you're eating.

3. **Size matters.** If you go to a restaurant and your portions are too large, cut them in half. You may find that by allowing yourself time to feel satiated, you won't even be hungry enough for the second half.

4. **Slow and steady.** Always try to eat slowly. It takes about twenty minutes for the signal indicating that you're full to go from your stomach to your brain. By slowing your pace, you'll avoid overeating. Try chewing each bite at least ten times.

5. **TV Time.** To minimize the amount of junk food you eat while watching the big game, measure low-fat snack foods such as pretzels and popcorn into serving sizes. You'll then be able to eyeball portion sizes and know when you're eating too much.

6. **Eat more often.** Aside from portion control, the frequency of your meals is also important. Simply put: more meals on smaller plates. We touched on the reasons for this earlier, when we discussed the *New Game Plan*. Just remember to eat five

small meals a day instead of three big ones. You won't be as hungry at each meal, so you'll be less likely to overeat. Plus, your body will metabolize the smaller meals more easily, which means you'll burn more calories and lose more weight.

7. **Stay well balanced.** I'm sure you've heard it said that you are what you eat. To some degree, it's true. However, if you simply stick to the new guidelines issued by the Institute of Medicine—50 percent carbohydrates, 30 percent protein, and 20 percent "good" fats, while also eating smaller, more frequent meals—the reality is that you don't need to diet. That's the Reality Diet in a nutshell (the obvious applies here regarding fried foods, excess alcohol, and desserts).

8. **Exercise often.** As outlined by the Institute of Medicine, everybody needs at least one hour of exercise every day. That can mean weight lifting, biking, running, walking—or even raking leaves. Perform high-intensity strength training workouts and aerobic exercise to maximize fat loss. Studies show that interval training (high-intensity exercise with little rest between sets) burns more calories than low- to moderate-intensity aerobic exercise, both during and after a workout.

## Busted Play #2

When Mrs. Right is pregnant, there is always the temptation to eat more—and more often. (There is also the temptation to tell her you're going to the store for milk, then empty your savings account, buy a motorcycle, ride it as far south as you can go without a visa, burn your fingerprints off with acid, and live out the rest of your days in a small fishing village, with no other responsibility than keeping yourself fed.) Anyway, if you're eating donuts and ice cream every night with Mrs. Right, no amount of portion control, meal timing, or exercise can combat fatty empty calories. And here's something else to be wary of: in the last trimester, many women grow lethargic. Mrs. Right sometimes has a mysterious way of transferring that feeling to us dads—making us less motivated to hit the gym.

> "My wife and I call the first three years of our children's lives the 'baby tunnel.' That's when you only have time to eat, sleep, and take care of the kids. If you're extra good, you get to take a shower. It's natural during the baby tunnel years to let yourself go a little."
>
> —KARL, a dad from Frisco, Texas

But it doesn't have to get to that point. Here are a couple of suggestions (some easier to follow than others):

- Say no to sweets.

- Keep your wife eating healthy, so you will have more choices.

- Stay away from buffets.

- Drink ten glasses of water a day.

- Don't eat after 8:00 P.M.

- Stick to an exercise program.

- Don't buy a motorcycle and ride it to Ecuador.

## Busted Play #3

In today's new (crappy) economy, just having a job can feel like a privilege, especially with a family to worry about and provide for. Under the *Original Game Plan*, it's okay to bounce from job to job. Don't like your boss? Quit. Don't like the hours? Quit.

Want more money? Find another job. I mean, what's the worst thing that could happen? If you run short on funds and need to make some lifestyle adjustments, you can always eat ramen noodles and crash on a buddy's couch.

But everything changes when you have your #1 draft pick and become a father. You are no longer responsible for just you. You can't just quit. You have to do everything in your power to keep your job—even if you don't like your boss, don't like the hours, and want a raise. Need motivation? Just go into your baby's room and watch him sleep. Or imagine you *and* your baby trying to crash on your buddy's couch.

Having a career and managing the family responsibilities that come with it can be very stressful. And that, too, is part of Busted Play #3.

Stress is the result of an experience that causes anger, frustration, or repulsion. Stress can be anything that creates tension and uncertainty. And take it from a dad and entrepreneur: children definitely create uncertainty, and work always creates tension. I can't tell you how many times I've come home from work, carrying a week's worth of tension in my shoulders, and, when my son runs headlong into my crotch and accidentally racks me, felt *very* uncertain that I had the willpower to keep from racking him back.

We feel stress because it was an evolutionary advantage. Imagine what would happen to the caveman who wandered across a saber-toothed tiger and didn't get a little stressed-out over the encounter. A relaxed caveman is a dead caveman. Stress is your body's fight-or-flight response.

Today, stress can still be a helpful tool. Your stress response might help you steer your car to avoid an accident or leap catlike into the air while pulling on your slacks when you're caught by the cleaning crew after hours in the copier room changing your secretary's toner. But today's stress, especially when caused by psychological or emotional factors, can be prolonged and may have damaging effects on your health.

One of the hormones released in the body during stressed or agitated states is cortisol. Cortisol is a steroid hormone made in the adrenal glands (neighbors of the kidneys). Among cortisol's important functions in the body are roles in the regulation of blood pressure and cardiovascular function, as well as regulation of the body's use of proteins, carbohydrates, and fats. And that's our big concern here. Fat. Cortisol leads to the release of fatty acids, an energy source from fat cells, for use by the muscles. Taken together, these energy-directing processes prepare us to deal with stressors and ensure that the brain receives adequate energy sources. However, when under stress, our bodies have a hard time converting fat into energy, so it's stored as fat. And that fat settles in as love handles, saddlebags, and man boobs. In fact, recent research findings suggest that men under high levels of stress were more likely to have extra fat around their midsections, which has been linked to heart disease, diabetes, hypertension, and certain types of cancer.

Literally, stress changes your body chemistry. And it can kill you.

Much of the problem stems from the way men's identities are so closely tied to work. Don't believe me? Next time you're at a cocktail party, pay attention to the first question men ask each other when they meet: "What do you do?" You *are* your job. Doctor, lawyer, whatever. That's how men define themselves. And all that does is create more stress. Because if you're identity is your work, then you certainly don't want to fail.

Has reading about all this stress stressed you out?

Don't fret. There are many simple and inexpensive ways to reduce your stress level. A good way to start is to cut out artificial stress reducers, such as alcohol or caffeine (do as I say, not as I do), which can mask symptoms and often make symptoms worse. Eat a well-balanced diet, which includes plenty of fruits and vegetables, as well as foods that are high in complex carbohydrates, moderate amounts of protein, and low in fat.

Aerobic activity, such as vigorous walking, is, in my opinion, the best way to reduce stress and improve overall quality of life (and you can do it with your family). Walk or do whatever type of exercise you feel comfortable with. You may prefer to join a health club. If you do join a health club, go often and make it your special time.

Go outdoors whenever possible. A little sunshine (a good source of vitamin A) and activity can dramatically reduce your stress level. Honestly, getting outside can enhance your entire outlook toward life. Your improved attitude will have a positive effect on everyone in your family and your circle of friends. Things that seem overwhelming will reveal themselves to be trivial matters, causing you to wonder what the predicament was. Not only will you be less stressed, you will be healthier, happier, and more energetic, ready to face whatever obstacles come your way.

Although we'll discuss in greater detail how to combat stress later, here are ten quick tips to help you tackle the stress monster:

1. **Breathe.** Breathe deeply, inhaling through your nose. Hold your breath for ten seconds, then exhale. You should feel your stomach expand with each breath. Sometimes closing your eyes or focusing on a pleasant place or a view helps.

2. **Pray or meditate.** Involve yourself in some form of spiritual activity. Set aside twenty to thirty minutes a day to commune with God or nature or your navel—whatever puts the universe in perspective for you.

3. **Stretch.** Get up and stretch to help break physical tension. Stand up, walk around your desk or the room. Gently roll

your head from side to side a few times. Roll your shoulders forward, then backward.

4. **Don't give in to the "gimmes."** Kids love to yell, "I want this, I want that!" It can wear parents down, but giving in to your child's every request can cause financial distress. It's okay to tell your child that something is too expensive. Tell him that even Santa Claus and Chanukah Harry have limited funds.

5. **Get eight hours.** Getting a good night's sleep is probably the easiest and most effective way for the body to reduce stress.

6. **Shed the superman mentality.** No one is perfect, so don't expect perfection from yourself *or* others.

7. **Turn off your cell phone (and/or pager and/or Blackberry) one day a week.** You'll be surprised how much people are always tugging on your cape.

8. **Learn to play again.** Just going to the batting cages or playing tag with your kids can be a good stress buster.

9. **Get a massage.** Aside from the medicinal benefits, a good hour-long massage can work wonders.

10. **Sex.** Have it. Not with your secretary. Unless she's really hot and can keep her mouth shut. Kidding, I'm just kidding.

Okay, so you've come to the realization that you're a Fat Daddy. And now you know that letting those love handles grow unchecked will not only make buying a swimsuit unpleasant but also can portend much more serious problems. In the next quarter, you will learn how to start to lose those love handles and butter gut—all while spending more quality time with your family.

Time to really study the *Keys to the Game*.

## PLAYBOOK NOTES: Penalty!
## Illegal Love Handles, Saddlebags,
## and Man Boobs

1. If you stand shirtless in front of a mirror and see breasts staring back at you, you can either shave them or face the fact that you have officially turned into a Fat Daddy.

2. Fat Daddies are not born, they are made over time; essentially, you are what you eat.

3. There are different body types that can accelerate Fat Daddy Syndrome.

4. There are many "busted plays" that aid in the development of Fat Daddies; there are also many solutions, like proper diet, exercise, and reducing stress.

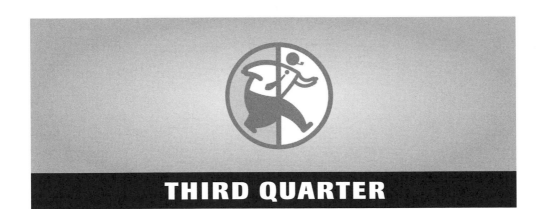

# The Keys to the Game

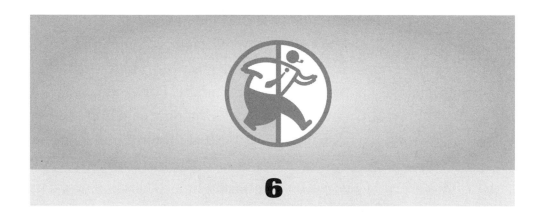

**6**

# The Training Table

"If he was married to Racquel Welch, he'd expect her to cook."

— former Dallas Cowboys' quarterback
DON MEREDITH on his coach, Tom Landry

## Food—The Foundation

Back in the day, before changing diapers and studying school districts, my friends and I would often challenge each other to perform gustatory feats of strength. Or, strengths of stupidity. It just depended on your perspective. Anyway, this would usually happen at a restaurant. We'd finish our meals, but there would be leftovers. A couple bites of a burger, a handful of cold French fries sitting under a helmet of congealed cheddar, a ramekin full of ranch dressing. Delicious stuff like that. Someone would say something like, "How much to drink the rest of that hot sauce?" Suddenly money was on the table—$15, more, perhaps, if we were really flush that night.

Sure, it doesn't seem like much now. But back when all your furniture was made from foam core and vinyl-covered reground polystyrene pellets, even a couple bucks was a lot of money. Still, that $15 bought us the joy of seeing a friend suffer. Plus, in the case of hot sauce, we not only got to see the suffering on the intake, we got to hear all about our pal's pain during the sauce's, well, outlet. I wasn't quite stupid enough to drink Tabasco, but I did accomplish a series of other gruesome gut-busting tasks. Indeed, I was known as the king of the food dare. In my proudest moment I downed 196 shrimp at an all-you-can-eat place for a payoff of just $12.75. You don't even want to know what that outlet was like. I'll just say too much fish oil is not pretty.

Those days, of course, are now gone. Ever since I became a Fat Daddy, my relationship with food has changed and eating, for me, is no longer a sport. I'm not alone in that. Or, at least, I shouldn't be alone.

But as we have discussed, we men go through life unprepared, and, what's worse, we're also *uninformed*. The chart below shows how most dads muddle through life on the food continuum.

| BABY BOY | GUY | HUSBAND | FATHER |
|---|---|---|---|
| | (Original Game Plan) eat whatever, whenever | (New Game Plan) eat on schedule | (New Teammates) eat whatever, whenever |
| Eats baby food | Eats cold pizza | Eats like a king | Eats baby food |

When we move on from the *Original Game Plan* and become Fat Daddies, the gustatory feats of strength may end, but the foods behind them don't. We're still eating cheese fries. We're just not agreeing to eat the leftover cheese fries that also happen to contain cigar (although, for $15 . . .). But there's a good reason to switch into a different dining defense. Food is the foundation of health. It matters what you eat, when you eat, and how you eat. Most important, it matters how *much* you eat. You can only lose weight if you consume fewer calories than you burn. To lose a pound of fat without changing your burn rate, you need to eliminate 3,500 calories a week from your diet. That's 500 calories a day. It doesn't actually matter where those calories come from—fats, carbs, protein, beer, whatever. To lose weight, you simply have to lose calories. However, to safely lose weight and get in better shape, you not only need to reduce your caloric intake, but you must do some form of exercise, too. We'll get down on the mat later, though.

It seems like women know a lot more about this stuff than men do. Pick up most women's magazines, and, besides "Sex Tricks He's Never Seen Before: The Outrageous Rock Technique," and "9 Steps to a Better Orgasm," you'll also find "27 Foods That Fight Fat" and "Beating the Belly Bulge: The Outrageous Rock Technique." But pick up most men's magazines and you'll find lots of pictures of hot chicks in lingerie. Just what in the hell does that teach you about improving your eating habits? Not a damn thing. Although, it certainly may improve your orgasm.

Anyway, how are we supposed to know that a bagel and jelly can actually make us fatter than two light waffles and syrup? How are we supposed know that buffets are bad? No one ever told us to eat *more* than three meals a day. How could we know that apples provide sustained, longer-term energy and help maintain stable blood sugar levels better than bananas because apples have a lower glycemic index? How are we supposed to know that there even is a glycemic index? We've got jobs to go to, for crying out loud. TV to watch. Porn to surf for. And the result: We're eating too much and too much of the wrong things.

It shouldn't be this way and it really doesn't have to. What, when, and how often we eat are not only critical to our own well-being, but our eating habits affect our families, too. As a father, you're a role model for the rest of your family. That's why you switched from doing beer bongs and keg stands at parties to slowly sipping Cosmos out of those cute martini glasses with the twisty bases. That's why you don't pile up your dirty boxers in front of the TV anymore. That's why, for freak's sake, you *dust*. But propping up a bag of cheesy puffs on your expanding gut while you watch the game—all the games, all day long—sets just as bad an example for your kids. When it comes to nutrition, studies have shown that parents do pass bad nutritional habits along to their kids. As a father, you have to stop that trend.

That's the reason I've made food the *foundation* of the Fat Daddy program. Without a strong grasp of good eating habits, dads will constantly fight the battle of the bulge and will eventually pass their own lumps of lard down to their children.

Another more recent study by the National Health and Nutrition Examination Survey (NHANES) indicate that an estimated 61 percent of U.S. adults are either overweight or obese, and four of the ten leading causes of death in the United States are directly linked to our diet. What's more, the bad eating habits that lead to such sad statistics seem to be cascading to our children. The Surgeon General's 2001 Call to Action against Obesity reported that 13 percent of young children and 14 percent of adolescents are overweight, with the number of overweight adolescents having tripled in two decades. *That's tripled in number*, not in size. Although that could have happened, too.

"An increasing number of kids are overweight, and if no intervention is made, 80 percent of them will stay overweight as adults," says Dr. Vincent Iannelli, a pediatrician who operates a website called KeepKidsHealthy.com. "This makes it important for the whole family to eat well and exercise together. Fathers (and mothers) have much more influence over their children than they generally believe, and if the parents are also involved in regular physical activity and are good role models, then their child is more likely to be active, too." The opposite is also true, he says. "If the parents are inactive and have a poor diet, then this gives the child little motivation to change his habits."

To compound the problem, kids used to get a lot of physical activity on playgrounds or exploring the neighborhood on foot. But today, kids spend their time in front of the TV or computer or standing around at a shopping mall. Even if they walk around the mall, they're stopping for a slice of pizza pie, or regular pie, or smoothies, or chocolate, or burgers, or fries, or maybe all of the above. Talk about your gustatory feats of strength. And the thing is all of that is turning us into a nation filled with Augustus Gloop look-alikes. Think about it. No? He's the fat, German kid from Willy Wonka. There you go.

Here are some more disturbing facts about our wide-body children:

- 50 percent do not get enough exercise to develop healthy heart and lung systems.

- 98 percent have at least one heart disease risk factor.

- 20 percent to 30 percent are obese.

- 75 percent eat too much dietary fat.

- Between 15 percent and 25 percent of schoolchildren in the United States are overweight, placing them at risk for heart disease, diabetes, and high blood pressure.

## We Had the Wrong Game Plan

So how did we get to be a nation of dumpy dads, morbidly obese moms, and Krispy Kreme kids? I'll blame the government. Those blockheads screw everything up. And what's with all these taxes? Okay, that's a different book.

But look at the famous Food Guide Pyramid developed by our pals in Washington at the United States Department of Agriculture (USDA). This cadre of farm bureaucrats has been the leading science on food in the United States for decades. We all learned about the food groups in school. We all bought into it.

No longer. The pyramid is now under fire, challenged by many of the leading authorities in health and nutrition. Tops on the list of pyramid bashers is Dr. Walter Willett and his colleagues at the Harvard School of Public Health. They've even developed their own Healthy Eating Pyramid. The main difference between the Healthy Eating Pyramid and the USDA pyramid is that the Harvard approach focuses on individual foods. Willett breaks up groups of fats or carbohydrates or proteins to highlight the best and worst sources of those nutrients. That may seem an obvious distinction, but it's a critical departure from the USDA's recommendations. Instead of directing people to the best fats, the most wholesome carbohydrates, and the most nutritious sources of protein, the USDA pyramid implies that all fats are dangerous and most carbs are safe. And if the past decade has taught us anything, it's that carbs can be as deadly as fats. Now, keep in mind that no single "nutritional pyramid" can perfectly suit every individual. Nutritional requirements depend on how efficient your metabolism is (metabolism is the rate at which your body will break down and use protein, carbohydrates, fats, vitamins, minerals, and so on). The faster your metabolism is, the easier it is to keep from gaining weight (usually). The slower your metabolism, the greater chance of your being overweight.

Most endomorphs have a slower metabolism than mesomorphs. But as I touched on earlier, the only way to change your metabolism is through proper diet and exercise. Combine that with the bad information we men usually operate with about food and it's easy to see why we're all growing Whopper waistlines.

# 1, 2, 3, Hike!

If the first *Key to the Game* is Food, simply remember the snap count —1, 2, 3—and you'll be fine.

1.  **How much:** portion control

2.  **How often:** frequency

3.  **What:** composition

## Portion Control

Anybody who has been on Weight Watchers not only knows the snap count, they know how to count points. The Weight Watchers' point system is all about portion control. As we discussed earlier, there has been much debate about calorie consumption, food combining, and the like (more about this in a minute). The *Fat Daddy* rule of thumb, er, make that thumb, fingers, and palm, is *if the amount of food on your plate is greater than the size of your outstretched hand, then your portion is too big.*

Unfortunately, portion sizes have been growing steadily in North America for the past thirty years, which can make it very difficult to figure out what an acceptable portion really looks like. While an average bagel weighed 2 to 3 ounces and contained 230 calories in the 1970s, it is now twice as large and contains about 550 calories.

In the 1970s, long before they were calling them "freedom fries," a serving of French fries consisted of about 30 fries and 450 calories. Today, some fast-food joints serve you about 50 fries containing a whopping 790 calories. The bottom line: If you don't put it on your plate, you won't have to worry about losing it later.

## Frequency

My mom used to tell me to eat three square meals a day. She also told me that if I masturbated I'd grow hair on my palms. (As it turns out, she was wrong on both counts. And I've researched enough on both to know that for sure—What? Like you haven't?)

Instead, eat four to six meals a day. Here's why:

- If you eat three meals a day, you're basically preparing your body for starvation. Yeah, starvation. Even if you eat small at all three meals. See, your brain releases chemicals after you eat to aid in digestion, absorption, and other metabolic processes between each meal. When you eat a large breakfast or lunch and then go three to five hours between feedings, your brain tells your body to slow down the process of converting food into energy. It stores the food instead, as if it was preparing for starvation. And it stores the food as fat. Tricky brain.

- When you only eat three large meals a day, your body also tends to regulate insulin poorly. Insulin is a hormone created in your pancreas that regulates your blood sugar levels. When your blood sugar levels spike because of the ingestion of lots of food at one time, or if you eat high glycemic foods like potatoes and pasta, your energy level drops and so does your body's ability to process that sugar. Hence, it stores it as fat for energy at a later date.

- When you load your body full of food, no matter how nutritious, you can only *properly* digest certain amounts of that food at each setting. As a result, even though the quality of the protein, carbohydrates, and fats might be acceptable, the *quantity* is not. Your body doesn't give you back the excess—it stores it as fat.

As I mentioned, the alternative is to eat more. Well, actually, less, but in more regular intervals. This will increase your energy level and your body's ability to burn fat more efficiently. Here's how:

■ More meals gives your body the ability to regulate insulin better. This keeps your energy levels more stable and makes it more efficient burning fat.

■ More meals tells your body that you are ingesting food on, well, a more frequent basis. It responds by burning that food as energy because it realizes that in two to three hours more food is on the way. This ability to speed up your metabolism directly increases the body's ability to burn more fat.

■ More meals keeps you from overeating. When you eat several small meals a day, you stabilize the body's cravings by not depriving it of nutrients and quality sustenance. If you eat two or three meals a day, you are probably overeating. If you find yourself famished between meals or "completely stuffed" after a meal, you need to cut down the portions and increase the frequency.

---

### SAMPLE DAY ANY DAD CAN DO

Approximately 2,000 calories, 50 percent carbohydrates,
35 percent protein, and 15 percent fat:

| WHEN | WHAT |
|---|---|
| *Breakfast* | 4 egg whites, oatmeal with walnuts and raisins, 10 oz. glass of orange juice |
| *Snack* | Orange |
| *Lunch* | Turkey sandwich on whole wheat bread, lettuce, tomato, low-fat mayo, mustard, and an apple |
| *Snack* | Cup of yogurt and a low-fat granola bar |
| *Dinner* | Chicken breast (or fish), brown rice, steamed green vegetables (broccoli, spinach, etc.) |
| *Snack* | Peanut butter sandwich on whole wheat, glass of low-fat milk or juice |

## Composition

As we discussed before, the healthiest diets should get about half of their calories from carbohydrates, one-quarter to one-third from fat, and the rest from protein. But before we start to dig into what's okay and what's not okay to eat, let's first take a look at the building blocks of the food we eat:

### *Carbohydrates (50 percent)*

Carbohydrates are the key to metabolic energy as well as to providing your body with the means to release the energy stored in fat and oxygen. The problem is that too many carbohydrates can make you fat! Just look at that Mario guy on the Food Network. See, your body can only properly digest a certain amount of carbohydrates at one sitting, and the rest are stored as fat. A good rule of thumb is not to exceed 30 to 50 grams of carbohydrates at one sitting unless you have just finished exercising (after exercising, your body needs carbohydrates to replenish the loss of glycogen from your working muscle tissue).

> **AUDIBLE**
>
> If you want to relax, or try to promote a sense of calm, eat more complex carbohydrates. Complex carbohydrates contain an amino acid called *tryptophan* that causes your brain to release a chemical called *serotonin*. When your brain releases serotonin, you usually become more relaxed and maybe even sleepy (listen up all of you type A's). So don't go hitting the pizza buffet before the big meeting!

The majority of carbohydrates are divided into three classes according to the amount of sugar units composing each carbohydrate molecule.

- **Monosaccharides.** A monosaccharide is a simple sugar. You will find these little sugars in most *fruits, honey, some sport drinks, and human breast milk*. Mmm. Breast milk.

■ **Disaccharides.** Disaccharides are "double" sugars made up of two monosaccharides bonded together. An example of disaccharides are *table sugar, lactose (milk), or maltose.*

■ **Polysaccharides.** Polysaccharides are complex sugars made up of many monosaccharides bonded together. These types of carbohydrates are also called *complex carbohydrates.* Complex carbohydrates are the most beneficial or "friendly carbohydrates" due to their chemical makeup. Since a complex (polysaccharide) carbohydrate is a group of carbohydrates bonded together, your body can much more easily use it for long-term energy.

### CARBOHYDRATE ALL-PROS
#### (Carbohydrate grams)

| MONOSACCHARIDES | DISACCHARIDES | POLYSACCHARIDES |
|---|---|---|
| Apple 20g (one medium) | Milk 2% 13g (medium cup) | Brown Rice 38g (cup) |
| Orange 20g (one medium) | Sugar 12g (teaspoon) | Whole Wheat Pasta 40g (cup) |
| Banana 25g (one medium) | Jelly 13g (teaspoon) | Potato with skin 30g (one medium) |
| Raisins 30g (large handful) | Syrup 13g (about a tablespoon) | Low-Fat Bran Muffin 45g |
| Honey 15g (teaspoon) | Cheese 3g (a slice) | Bagel 30g (one medium) |

Above figures are averages for each selected food. Portion size may minimally vary.

Another important note about carbohydrates is their *glycemic index.* The glycemic response of a food is a measure of the food's ability to regulate blood sugar. The glycemic response is also influenced by the carbohydrate's fiber content, fat content, and the way it's prepared. Highly glycemic carbohydrates are best consumed during and after exercise. They enter the bloodstream quickly and are readily available for fueling exercising muscles. Low glycemic carbohydrates enter the bloodstream slowly and are best eaten before exercise. They provide sustained longer-term energy and help maintain stable blood sugar levels during extended exercise periods—say, greater than one hour, or just about as long as it takes you to have sex. Hah. Now *that's* funny. The table below shows some examples of foods and their glycemic index number. Remember, higher is better during or right after exercise, and a lower index number is better at least an hour or earlier before exercise. If you don't exercise, stick with the lower index foods.

| HIGHLY GLYCEMIC FOODS | | MODERATELY GLYCEMIC FOODS | | LOW GLYCEMIC FOODS | |
|---|---|---|---|---|---|
| Glucose | 100 | Orange Juice (medium glass) | 57 | Apple (one medium) | 36 |
| Baked Potato (medium) | 85 | White Rice (one cup) | 56 | Pear (one medium) | 36 |
| Corn Flakes (bowl) | 84 | Popcorn (large portion) | 55 | Skim Milk (small glass) | 32 |
| Cheerios (bowl) | 74 | Corn (one ear) | 55 | Green Beans (one cup) | 30 |
| Honey (tablespoon) | 73 | Brown Rice (one cup) | 55 | Lentils, Beans (one cup) | 29 |

| HIGHLY GLYCEMIC FOODS | | MODERATELY GLYCEMIC FOODS | | LOW GLYCEMIC FOODS | |
|---|---|---|---|---|---|
| Watermelon (large slice) | 72 | Sweet Potato (one medium) | 54 | Grapefruit (one medium) | 25 |
| Bagel (one medium) | 72 | Banana (one medium) | 50 | Grains, Barley (one cup) | 25 |

### *Protein (35 percent)*

Proteins are the most fundamental constituents of living matter. Proteins function as the major structural and functional component of every living cell in our bodies.

Not only are proteins a necessity for the function of cells, they are also the main building blocks for muscle tone, growth, hair luster, nail strength, and hormone balance. All foods contain some type of protein, but the amount and quality of protein vary greatly. Meat, fish, poultry, legumes, eggs, nuts, soy, and most dairy products are all high in protein. Vegetables and grains contain proteins, but to a much lesser extent.

> **AUDIBLE**
>
> If you are going to an important meeting or have to be extremely alert and responsive, eat *primarily protein.* Why? Most proteins contain an amino acid called *tyrosine.* Tyrosine causes the release of several chemicals in your brain, mainly *norepinphine* and *dopamine.* These two chemicals cause you to be more alert and sharp.

The easiest way to make sure you get enough protein each day is to try to have some form of meat, fish, poultry, legumes, eggs, nuts, soy, or dairy products at every meal. As a rule of thumb, the average

*Fat Daddy* should have about .5 to .75 grams of protein per pound of body weight.

**Example:** *170 lb. Man × .5 = 82.5 grams of protein/day.*

| HIGH PROTEIN FOODS | (GRAMS) |
|---|---|
| Fish (medium portion) | 30+ |
| Pork (one chop) | 30 |
| Lamb (medium shank) | 27 |
| Chicken breast (skinless) | 22 |
| Legumes (one cup) | 20 |
| Oats (one cup) | 18 |
| Yogurt (low/nonfat cup) | 16 |
| Cottage Cheese (one cup) | 12 |
| Egg whites (1 egg) | 4 |
| *Figures are averages for each selected food. Portion size may minimally vary.* | |

### Fats (15 percent)

Despite what we've been taught our entire lives, fat is not completely bad for you. Nothing that tastes that good could be all bad, right? The thing is that not all fats are created equal. But they are a very important part of what we should eat. Fats occur naturally in food and play an important role in nutrition. Fats and oils provide a concentrated source of energy for the body. Fats are used to store energy in the body, insulate body tissues, and transport fat-soluble vitamins through the blood. They also play an important role in food preparation by enhancing food flavor, adding mouth-feel—yes, mouth-feel—and making baked products chewy and tender. But ever since word got out that diets high in fat are related to heart disease (something that is enemy No. 1 when it comes to knocking off us men), things have become more complicated. Experts tell us there are several different kinds of fat, some of them worse for us than others. In addition to saturated, monounsaturated, and polyunsaturated fats, there are triglycerides, trans fatty acids, and omega-3 and omega-6 fatty acids.

Almost every day there are newspaper reports of new studies or recommendations about what fats to eat or what fats not to eat: Lard is bad, olive oil is good, and margarine is better for you than butter. Or, then again, maybe it's not.

Despite most dietary guidelines, adults in North America consume about 36 percent of their daily energy as fatty acids, with total intakes ranging from 65 to 100 grams per day. That may not be all that bad, as long as you stay with the "good fats."

### The Good Fats

- **Polyunsaturated fatty acids** are found mainly in vegetable oils such as safflower, sunflower, corn, flaxseed, and canola oils. Polyunsaturated fats are also the main fats found in seafood. They are liquid or soft at room temperature. Specific polyunsaturated fatty acids, such as linoleic acid and alpha-linolenic acid, are called essential fatty acids. They are necessary for cell structure and making hormones. Essential fatty acids must be obtained from foods we choose.

- **Omega-3 fats** are found in so-called "fatty fish" such as salmon, halibut, mackerel, or sardines. These members of the polyunsaturated fat family seem to provide special protection for the heart, especially abnormal heart rhythms that are responsible for sudden death syndrome (like that of Korey Stringer of the Minnesota Vikings in 2001).

■ **Monounsaturated fatty acids** are found mainly in vegetable oils such as canola, olive, and peanut oils. They are liquid at room temperature.

### The Bad Fats

■ **Saturated fats** are found chiefly in animal sources such as meat and poultry, whole or reduced-fat milk, and butter. Some vegetable oils like coconut, palm kernel oil, and palm oil are saturated. Saturated fats are usually solid at room temperature.

■ **Trans fatty acids** are formed when vegetable oils are processed into margarine or shortening. Sources of trans fats in the diet include snack foods and baked goods made with partially hydrogenated vegetable oil or vegetable shortening. Trans fatty acids also occur naturally in some animal products such as dairy products.

## Diet Reality and the "Reality Diet"

Now that we have barked out the snap count on the big three—carbs, proteins, and fats—it's time to take the diet ball and run. But before we look at the ten best ways to score, I wanted to give you an objective look at what other diet and eating plans prescribe.

### The Atkins Diet, Robert C. Atkins, M.D.

■ **The details:** Carbs, not fat, are the culprit behind obesity, according to Atkins, based on the premise that heavy carb consumption causes you to store more food as fat. If you deprive the body of carbs, it's forced to burn fat reserves for energy. The solution: a high-fat, low-carbohydrate diet. It allows no more carbohydrates than the equivalent of two cups of salad a day for the first two weeks.

- **Pros:** Good for quick weight loss. The fatty meals leave dieters feeling full and satisfied.

- **Cons:** Saturated fats increase the risk of heart disease. Cutting out fresh produce can deprive the body of vitamins and beneficial plant chemicals. Plus, just try to eat at a restaurant with an Atkins dieter. Two words: High maintenance.

## The Zone, Barry Sears, Ph.D.

- **The details:** Based on the balanced consumption of nutrients. Your daily intake should consist of 30 percent protein, 30 percent fat, and 40 percent carbohydrates. (30 + 30 + 40 = 100. See, more math.) This ratio supposedly stimulates the ideal production of insulin, which in turn may encourage weight loss and a host of other health and emotional benefits.

- **Pros:** Encourages lean protein sources that are low in saturated fat. Not as carbo-restrictive as Atkins.

- **Cons:** The strict balance of food groups makes it tough to figure out portions. Critics say it's simply a calorie-restriction diet, the insulin theory aside.

## Eat More, Weigh Less, Dean Ornish, M.D.

- **The details:** A largely vegetarian diet in which only 10 percent of your calories should come from fat. The high-fiber plan favors vegetables, beans, whole grains, and fruit, which can be eaten until you feel full. Low-fat dairy products like skim milk and nonfat yogurt and egg whites can be eaten in moderation.

Dieters should avoid meats, oils, olives, and sugar as much as possible.

■ **Pros:** Studies have shown that Ornish's low-fat diet can reverse the risk of heart disease. Overall, a great program (okay, full disclosure: Dean's dad was my orthodontist, so I'm a little biased).

■ **Cons:** His fat ban may be too broad. And if you eat virtually all vegetables, how long will it be before you're wearing clothes made from hemp?

### The Blood Type Diet, Peter J. D'Adamo, M.D.

■ **The details:** According to D'Adamo, you should choose certain foods and avoid others depending on your blood type. If you eat the wrong foods, the effect on your body is similar to receiving a transfusion of the wrong type of blood. The recommended daily number of calories varies.

■ **Pros:** All blood types are encouraged to consume many servings of fruits and vegetables. Sources of lean protein are also recommended. This plan can be easier to follow than diets that severely restrict calories.

■ **Cons:** D'Adamo's claim isn't supported by scientific research and is widely criticized as being based on false assumptions. So there's that.

### Pritikin Diet, Robert Pritikin

■ **The details:** This diet restricts fat intake to 10-15 percent of total calories in an attempt to curb the "fat instinct," which Pritikin claims is a biological drive to avoid exercise and eat too much high-fat food. The consumption of complex, fibrous carbohydrates, such as fruits and veggies, is encouraged.

- **Pros:** Lean cuts of meat are recommended, which reduces calories and the risk of heart disease.

- **Cons:** Most men won't feel satisfied for a long period of time after eating a meal containing such a small amount of fat. This may lead to overeating. And that leads to being fat. And being fat is kind of, like, the whole thing you're trying to avoid.

### The Caveman Diet, Ray Audette

- **The details:** According to Audette, modern processed foods such as wheat and grains are to be blamed for obesity. He also opines that the caveman stayed lean thanks to a diet composed of lean meat, fish, nuts, seeds, berries, and fresh fruits and veggies.

- **Pros:** The recommended "whole" foods contain more vitamins and nutrients than processed foods. This program may be easier for men to follow than calorie-restricted diets.

- **Cons:** His theory isn't supported by any research. Then again, it is a hit with that Rob Becker guy. If you don't get that, look it up.

### The Cabbage Soup Diet, Margaret Danbrot

- **The details:** This word-of-mouth diet was finally put into writing by Danbrot, who claims that you can lose up to twenty pounds in seven days by consuming a vegetable-based soup (cabbage, onions, peppers, tomatoes, celery, and onion soup mix) and one other food.

- **Pros:** Rapid weight loss.

■ **Cons:** The weight loss, which is due to loss of water or lean body tissue, is temporary. It can also lead to side effects such as nausea and lightheadedness. There's also the gas. Oh, sweet fancy Moses, the gas.

### The Calorie Restriction (or Starvation) Diet, Scientists at MIT

■ **The details:** By drastically reducing a person's calorie intake to under 950 calories per day, the calorie restrictive diet appears to create biochemical changes that have a more profound effect on lifespan than simply avoiding diseases caused by excess fat.

■ **Pros:** Rapid weight loss, possible longer lifespan.

■ **Cons:** Extreme hunger pangs, lightheadedness, weakness. And, of course, starvation.

Many of these diets and programs work for many people. But most dads need a simple play they can run many times in every game for the rest of their life, not just when they need three yards for a first down in the fourth quarter of the Super Bowl. Basically what I'm trying to say is that eating right and dieting are not the same thing. One is a lifestyle; the later is a temporary change in behavior.

I call the Fat Daddy lifestyle plan the **Reality Diet**.

## The Reality Diet, Lawrence Schwartz, R.F.D. (Recovering Fat Daddy)

■ **The details:** Closely mirrors the National Institute of Health's 50 percent carbs, 30 percent protein, 20 percent fat per meal breakdown. Stresses **portion** size and meal **frequency** but doesn't restrict all foods. Exercise plays a critical role.

■ **Pros:** Easy to follow, reinforces the obvious, heart healthy, and practical.

■ **Cons:** A svelte, handsome body that the ladies will kill for. So watch out for your wife!

## The Reality Diet—Ten Key Plays

1. Never eat more on your plate than your outstretched hand.

2. Eat four to six small meals per day.

3. Always eat *protein* and some type of *vegetable* at every *major* meal (breakfast, lunch, and dinner).

4. Lighten up on breads, potatoes, and pastas.

5. Always drink at least eight glasses of water per day.

6. Never have more than two cups of coffee or two diet drinks per day.

7. Limit fried foods to only once per week (this includes chips).

8. If you drink alcohol, have one glass of water after every alcoholic drink.

9. Never eat after 8:00 P.M. (or at least three hours before bedtime).

10. When dining out: (a) always ask for grilled, baked, or steamed; (b) ask for dressings on the side—and only use half; and (c) refuse the bread.

## Fat Daddy WARNING!!

Despite the hype, a high-protein, low-carbohydrate diet is NOT recommended:

- **It is inadequate in major nutrients (i.e., carbohydrates and fiber) as well as micronutrients** (i.e., many vitamins, minerals, antioxidants and phytochemicals).

- **It promotes water (not fat) loss.** It gives one a false sense of weight loss due to an immediate loss of body fluid. May also cause excessive potassium loss, electrolyte imbalance, and dehydration. Rarely is weight loss permanent.

- **It may cause ketosis.** High-protein, low-carbohydrate diets result in the formation of ketones (vs. glucose) as a source of fuel. Ketones are formed and released into the bloodstream resulting in ketosis (a fasting type state). Ketosis suppresses appetite, may cause muscle breakdown, causes nausea, dehydration, headaches, lightheadedness, irritability, bad breath (no kidding), and potential kidney problems. In pregnancy, ketosis may cause fetal abnormalities or death.

- **Will slow your metabolism.** By reducing carbohydrates you will see a drop of body weight and body fat. However, if you drop them too low while exercising, you could alter your body's T3 levels. T3 is an active thyroid molecule that helps regulate your metabolic rate. Diets low in carbohydrates tend to cause a reduction of T3, which in turn can slow down your metabolic rate. This is particularly true for people who undereat and overexercise.

- **It is often low in fiber,** causing constipation and possibly increasing one's risk for colon cancer.

- **It often contains higher than recommended amounts of cholesterol and saturated fat,** increasing one's risk of heart disease and cancer. Excessive red meat consumption has been linked to colon and prostate cancer.

■ **It may raise uric acid levels,** increasing one's risk of gout.

■ **Excessive protein may leach calcium from the bones,** increasing one's risk of osteoporosis.

■ **No controlled studies prove its safety or effectiveness,** unlike the dietary recommendations made by the AHA and ADA.

Now that you know which diets to stay away from, and you understand the foundation of the Reality Diet, let's apply the theory to real-life situations that a dad may encounter.

| BREAKFAST/BRUNCH | |
| --- | --- |
| **FIRST DOWN** | **LOSS OF DOWN** |
| Egg whites or Egg Beaters | Whole eggs |
| Egg white omelet | Eggs Benedict |
| Whole wheat toast without butter (honey is okay) | Toast with butter |
| Oatmeal | Pancakes |
| Whole grain cereal | Cereals that are full of sugar |
| Fruit or fruit juice | Chocolate milk |
| Skim milk | Whole milk |
| Fat-free or nonfat yogurt | Regular yogurt |
| Bagel without cream cheese | Bagel with cream cheese |
| Jelly/jam/fat-free butter | Butter |
| Coffee/tea | Café latte or cappuccino |
| Granola | Bacon |

## ITALIAN FOOD

| FIRST DOWN | LOSS OF DOWN |
|---|---|
| Red sauce/wine sauce/marinara/lemon | Cream sauce/cheese/Alfredo/bacon |
| Focaccia bread | Garlic bread (it's loaded with butter!) |
| Grilled/baked | Sautéed/fried |
| Picatta | Parmigiana |
| Primavera | Lasagna |

## MEXICAN FOOD

| FIRST DOWN | LOSS OF DOWN |
|---|---|
| Corn tortillas | Flour tortillas |
| Marinated | Fried |
| Beans | Refried beans |
| Picante sauce | Con queso |
| Grilled | Stuffed with cheese |
| Chili | Guacamole |
| Rice | Chips |
| Enchilada sauce | Sour cream |
| Fresh vegetables | Fried veggies |
| Light beer | Margarita (lots more calories) |

| ASIAN FOOD | |
|---|---|
| **FIRST DOWN** | **LOSS OF DOWN** |
| Simmered | Fried |
| Grilled | "Crispy" |
| Steamed | Golden |
| Braised | Breaded |
| Szechwan | Peanut sauce |
| Sushi | Curry |
| Bean curd or tofu | Tempura |
| Spring rolls | Egg rolls |
| Sashimi | Sweet and sour dishes |
| Thai | Stir fried in oil |
| Hot and sour soup | Egg drop soup |

| SEAFOOD | |
|---|---|
| **FIRST DOWN** | **LOSS OF DOWN** |
| Grilled | Fried |
| Poached | Sautéed |
| Baked | Stuffed |
| Blackened | Lemon butter |
| Cajun | Au gratin |
| Wine sauce | Cream sauce |
| Herbs | Hollandaise |
| En brochette | Crab Louis |

| FAST FOOD | |
|---|---|
| **FIRST DOWN** | **LOSS OF DOWN** |
| Grilled chicken | Burgers |
| Bean burritos (no cheese please) | Taco salads (they can contain up to 40g of fat!) |
| Rotisserie chicken | Fried chicken |
| Baked potato (no cheese or sour cream) | French fries |
| Pretzels | Chips |
| Turkey/chicken sub | Anything fried |
| Salad bar (no pasta or other foo foo stuff) | Hot dogs |
| Baked fish | Fried fish |
| Cookies | Hot apple pie |
| Diet soda or water | Milk shake |

| SNACKS | |
|---|---|
| **FIRST DOWN** | **LOSS OF DOWN** |
| Pretzels | Chips |
| Baked chips | Dips |
| Almonds | Peanuts or pistachios |
| Fat-free dips | Hot wings |
| Carrot or celery sticks | Candy/cookies |
| Turkey squares | Anything fried |

## The Cholesterol Battle

Dads love to talk about their battle with cholesterol. Really. You can't get them to shut up about it. Blah, blah, cholesterol, blah. Which cholesterol is good? Which cholesterol is bad? How do I get it? How do I get rid of it? Yada, yada, yada.

To be sure, it is a confusing subject even for us dads who understand the differences between light beer and regular beer. So let's break down the cholesterol conundrum nice and slow.

A person's cholesterol "number" refers to the total amount of cholesterol in the blood (cholesterol is a fat carried around in our body in combination with proteins called "lipoproteins"). There are two types of cholesterol: low-density lipoprotein ("LDL") and high-density lipoprotein ("HDL"). A high level of LDL cholesterol in the blood increases the risk of fatty deposits forming in the arteries, which in turn increases the risk of a heart attack. Thus, LDL cholesterol has been dubbed "bad" cholesterol. On the other hand, an elevated level of HDL cholesterol seems to remove these fatty deposits (known as plaque) and has a protective

> ### GOAL LINE DEFENSE
> - Eating too many foods high in saturated fat is BAD.
> - Trans fatty acids are BAD.
> - Eating foods high in monounsaturated fat is GOOD.
> - Eating polyunsaturated fats is GOOD.

effect against heart disease. For this reason, HDL cholesterol is often called "good" cholesterol. Repeat that: LDL is bad. HDL is good. And puppies are adorable.

Doctors recommend that total blood cholesterol be kept below 200 while the average level in adults in this country is 205 to 215. The National Institute of Health further breaks down that number and recommends that individuals should have an HDL cholesterol level of more than 35 and an LDL cholesterol level of less than 130 to minimize the risk of heart disease. But, of course, the higher your HDL and the lower your LDL, the better.

## Tips for the Journeyman
## (The Traveling Fat Daddy)

Eating on the road can be a recipe for disaster. Just think of all the fat, sodium, and empty calories that are lurking in your neighborhood convenience store or vending machine. And we're not even going to talk about those hot dogs. But just because you're traveling doesn't mean you can't stick with the plan. A business trip is not an excuse to eat the wrong foods. It just takes a little more effort to stay on plan, but not much. I'm confident that anyone and everyone can commit to eat right on the road. I have been traveling upwards of three days per week for ten years. If I can do it, so can you. Here's how:

### "If by Land"

Stop off at any grocery store.

- Stock up on water-packed tuna or low-sodium turkey breast.

- Pick up some apples, oranges, carrots, and even broccoli.

- Pick up some rice cakes, fat-free crackers, or some whole wheat bread.

You don't need a fancy place in order to eat a nutritious, filling meal. Be resourceful. Be creative. But most of all be committed to your *own* health. If you're in the car, get a cheap cooler and pack it with food. If your hotel has a small refrigerator, load it up. Just don't let your job or environment make you fat.

**"If by Air"**

Some airline meals have as much as 40 grams of fat! So when you or your travel agent makes your plane reservation, ask the airline for a *low-fat* or *low-sodium* meal. Their selections range from turkey pita sandwiches to shrimp cocktail. Also, when traveling by plane, drink plenty of water. The cabin pressure tends to cause dehydration.

# Cold Beer Here

Tastes great. Less filling. Unless, of course, by "filling" you mean "calories" and then beer is plenty filling. Because the calories contain virtually no nutrition. They're what we call "empty," but they can still make you fat. So here's how you should handle drinking: Go ahead and drink. No, don't. No, do. I drink sometimes and then I may not for months. So, my advice is, drink smart. Know what you're consuming and how to keep it from consuming you.

The bad news is that alcohol consumption is the biggest drug problem in the United States today. Its abuse can affect everyone in a family. The good news is that there are health benefits to drinking alcohol, too. Alcohol helps your heart and arteries (the ethanol elevates HDL cholesterol). Even a study in the *New England Journal of Medicine* found that one to seven alcoholic beverages per week can significantly reduce middle-aged and older men's risk of having a stroke. However, the opposite was found to be true for heavy drinkers. More than five glasses of alcohol daily increased overall risk of stroke by 64 percent. Heavy drinking increased the risk of strokes by 69 percent, compared with teetotalers.

So abuse is bad, but consumption is not. Still, as I said before, be smart, especially if you are trying to lose those love handles. Alcohol can add hundreds of calories to your daily diet without adding any appreciable amounts of vitamins or minerals. And that can make the difference between weight loss, maintaining your current weight, or gaining weight. A single glass of beer or wine can contain 100 calories. Having a few drinks three or four nights a week could be adding 1,000 unforeseen calories to your diet per week. Alcohol also acts as an appetite stimulant, leading you to eat or crave foods that are not within your weight-loss plan. Potato skins, for instance. Or cheese fries. With extra ranch, of course. What's worse, the liver diverts those empty calories into making fat, which is then stored in the liver before being carried away to permanent storage sites (read: man boobs).

Let's make the bottom line here extra clear just in case you've been drinking your way through this section. Alcohol can be good for adults in small amounts. Moderate drinking appears to lower the risk of heart disease, stroke, and other diseases. But alcohol can be very dangerous, so drink responsibly—within your goals for your own appearance, and within the law.

## Extra Point

It's obvious, if you're a Fat Daddy trying to lose his love handles, you've probably been avoiding burgers and fries. Although this is definitely a good start, there are many other foods out there that may seem "safe" when, in fact, they are actually very high in calories or fat. Don't be fooled; the following ten foods are actually not as good for you as you may have thought.

1. **Frozen yogurt.** In this case, you really have to read the label. While some brands are relatively low-calorie, others have even more calories than light ice cream. Thanks to a ton of added sugar, some premium brands pack up to 185 calories per half-cup.

*Two-point conversion: Make sure that no matter what kind of low-fat frozen dessert you choose, it has no more than 120 calories per half-cup.*

2. **Fat-free snacks.** Most of these seemingly healthy snacks have almost no fiber and are easy to eat in huge quantities because they're not satisfying. Many even have more calories per serving than the regular version in order to compensate for the lack of tasty fat. The result? You could end up consuming a lot more calories than if you just ate a reasonable portion of the high-fat food you were craving in the first place.

   *Two-point conversion: Simply choose a healthier snack such as veggies and fat-free dip or buy fat-free snacks in small quantities in order to avoid stuffing your pie hole.*

3. **Popcorn.** At the movies, you should definitely skip the popcorn. The smallest child-size bag, without the extra butter, packs up to 300 cals and 20 grams of fat. The microwave kind can be even worse; many brands have almost 400 cals and 26 fat grams per bag.

   *Two-point conversion: Air pop it or choose a reduced-fat microwave version. If you wish, season with garlic chili powder or sprinkle on some Tabasco sauce to add flavor.*

4. **Olive oil.** With less than two grams of saturated fat per tablespoon, olive oil is healthier than most vegetable oils and it may even reduce your risk of heart disease. However, keep in mind that it's still oil; one tablespoon contains 120 cals and 14 grams of fat, so go easy if you don't want to sabotage your diet.

   *Two-point conversion: Use only a small amount for cooking or try olive oil cooking spray. A one-second spray has only seven calories and less than one gram of fat.*

5. **Frozen diet meals.** They may be convenient, nutritious, and low in fat and calories, but most are full of sodium, which can raise both your blood pressure and risk of heart attack. Plus, the minuscule portions are not satisfying enough for most men, which can lead to overeating later.

   *Two-point conversion: Don't eat more than one prepared food that contains more than 600 milligrams of sodium per day. And look for the word "healthy" on labels; it can't be used if the food has more than 480 milligrams of sodium per serving.*

6. **Protein bars.** These were designed for hard-core athletes, so drop that bar if you're not one of them. Although they're not bad for you, they can contain up to 300 calories and more protein than you need in an entire day. Now is that really necessary?

   *Two-point conversion: Before you work out, have a piece of whole wheat toast with a tablespoon of peanut butter (180 calories) or a fat-free yogurt and half a banana (220 calories).*

7. **Fast-food grilled chicken.** Although grilled is definitely better than fried, most fast-food grilled chicken sandwiches are full of fat due to all the cheese and creamy toppings they're smothered in. For example, Burger King's BK Broiler chicken sandwich contains 530 calories and 26 fat grams.

   *Two-point conversion: Ask them to hold the sauce or simply opt for a healthier restaurant. A good choice is Subway, whose six-inch chicken sub has only 332 calories and 6 grams of fat.*

8. **Granola.** Granola may seem "natural" and healthy, but that doesn't mean it won't make you fat. Most granola bars con-

tain tons of hydrogenated oil, which means that two-thirds of a cup add up to about 380 calories and 20 grams of fat.

*Two-point conversion: The good thing about granola is that it's a great source of fiber, with more than 8 grams per serving. Fortunately, there are many other sources of fiber to choose from, such as a satisfying bowl of instant oatmeal. (Tip: Stick to the individual packets, which are a good serving size.) Or you can try low-fat granola with fruit and skim milk, which will save you around 17 grams of fat and 170 calories per serving.*

9. **Tuna salad sandwich.** The tuna itself is very healthy; besides the fact that it is low in calories and fat, it is a great source of protein and healthy omega-3 fatty acids. The problem with this fishy favorite is all the mayo that usually goes into it. Get this: A typical tuna sandwich at a restaurant contains up to a whopping 720 cals and 43 grams of fat.

    *Two-point conversion: Try to avoid it altogether when eating out because the mayo is often already mixed in, which makes it difficult to ask for less. At home, use fat-free mayo and whole wheat bread to save up to 180 calories and 18 grams of fat.*

10. **Salad.** You're probably wondering how fattening lettuce could possibly be. While it's true that most vegetables contain few calories, the culprit in most salads is the dressing. In fact, if your salad is drowned in creamy ranch or blue cheese dressing, you could be getting as many calories as you would with a huge plate of fries. Believe it or not, the most popular salad in the United States, chicken Caesar, is also the most fattening. According to the Center for Science in the Public Interest (CSPI), a typical chicken Caesar salad contains an unbelievable 660 cals and 46 grams of fat.

*Two-point conversion: Use fat-free dressing at home.*
*When eating out, ask for dressing on the side and use the*
*"fork method." Dip your fork into the dressing, shake the*
*fork, then spear the salad; you'll save up to 20 grams of fat*
*. . . eat better and feel better.*

## PLAYBOOK NOTES: The Training Table

1. Food is the foundation to good health.

2. Portion size, frequency, and quality of food are keys to a good nutritional program.

3. Diets are bad; you DIE ON IT.

4. Try to stick to a 50 percent carbohydrate, 35 percent protein, and 15 percent fat diet.

5. Doctors recommend that total blood cholesterol be kept below 200.

6. Alcohol can be good for adults in small amounts and appears to lower the risk of heart disease, stroke, and other diseases.

7. Watch out for fast-food fumbles.

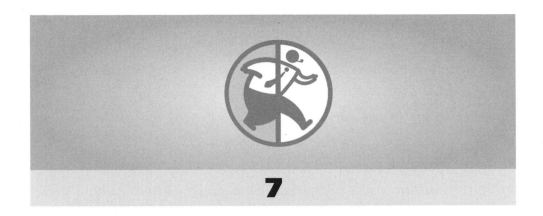

# 7

# Now a Word from Our Supplement Sponsor

"Spectacular achievements are always preceded by unspectac- ular preparation."

—ROGER STAUBACH, former Dallas Cowboy Hall of Fame quarterback

## The Missing Player

If you're not eating a well-balanced diet, you may be gaining weight but you're losing something else—essential nutrients. So what? A lack of nutrients leads to fatigue, depression, increased irritability, mood swings, loss of bone density, decrease in lean muscle, anemia, low blood levels of iron, and chronic illnesses. But don't start writing your eulogy just yet. Many foods are fortified with a percentage of the recommended daily allowance of vitamins and minerals. However, if you are a typical dad who is overworked, overstressed, and undersexed (who ain't?), your body needs even more nutrients than that to function well. Dietary supplements can come off the bench and help out. They're the player you're missing.

Dietary supplements are widely available through many commercial sources including health food stores, grocery stores, pharmacies, and by mail and come in many forms including tablets, capsules, powders, geltabs, extracts, and liquids. Historically in the United States, the most prevalent type of dietary supplement was a multivitamin/mineral tablet or capsule that was available in pharmacies by prescription or over the counter. However, a wide array of supplement products are available. They include vitamin, mineral, other nutrients, and botanical supplements as well as ingredients and extracts of animal and plant origin.

Supplements can have many valuable benefits:

■ Men who have trouble conceiving may get a boost from nutritional supplements that increase sperm count. A new study published in the March 2002 issue of *Fertility and Sterility* found a combination of folic acid and zinc supplements increased sperm count by 74 percent in men with fertility problems.

■ *The Journal of Cancer* (November 1, 1999) found that men with low levels of beta-carotene in their blood can reduce their risk of prostate cancer by as much as 32 percent by taking beta-carotene supplements every other day. That's big, because the American Cancer Society estimates that nearly every year 200,000 men will be diagnosed with prostate cancer and 40,000 will die.

■ In two separate studies, European scientists at the University of Vienna and the University of Innsbruck have found that dietary supplements—primarily containing vitamin E and fish oil supplements such as marine omega-3 fatty acids—can improve heart artery function and in some cases decrease heart disease.

What's more, many multivitamin and mineral supplements contain important antioxidants. Antioxidants prevent oxidation by free radicals. Really, they do. Let's say that in English. When cells are oxidized by these free radicals, they age prematurely. Or they may mutate into cancer cells. Your food can help that bad stuff to happen if it contains certain oxidants. Margarine, for instance, is an oxidant. And data shows there is a direct relationship between the advent of margarine use and the increase in cancer cases in the United States. Antioxidants can fight the bad stuff, though. A slew of research shows antioxidants are, in fact, among the most critical nutrients in the prevention of illness and they can help increase longevity. So get some supplements. Like, now.

---

### THE FAT DADDY SUPPLEMENT ALL PROS
TIP: You can get all of these in a good multivitamin.

| WHAT | WHY | WHERE TO GET IT | RECOMMENDATION FOR MEN AGES 11 AND UP |
|---|---|---|---|
| Vitamin A | Important for good vision, especially at night, immunity, reproduction, and the growth and maintenance of cells of the skin, gastrointestinal tract, and other mucus membranes | Fortified milk, eggs, liver, cheese, leafy green vegetables (e.g., spinach, kale, turnip greens, collards, romaine lettuce), broccoli, dark orange fruits and vegetables | 1000 micrograms RE/day (equivalent to about 5000 IU) |

*(Continued)*

| WHAT | WHY | WHERE TO GET IT | RECOMMENDATION FOR MEN AGES 11 AND UP |
|------|-----|-----------------|----------------------------------------|
| Vitamin A (Continued) | | (e.g., apricots, carrots, pumpkin, sweet potatoes, papaya, mango, cantaloupe), red bell peppers | |
| B-1 | Important for producing energy from carbohydrates, and for proper nerve function | Pork, liver, legumes, nuts, whole grain or enriched breads and cereals | 1.2 milligrams/day |
| B-2 | Contributes to energy production | Lean meats, yogurt, milk, cheese, eggs, broccoli, whole grain or enriched breads and cereals | 1.7 milligrams/day |
| B-3 (also called niacin) | Contributes to energy production; important for health of skin, digestive tract, and nervous system | Protein-rich foods, including milk, eggs, meat, poultry, fish, nuts, enriched cereals and grain products | 20 milligrams/day |

| WHAT | WHY | WHERE TO GET IT | RECOMMENDATION FOR MEN AGES 11 AND UP |
|---|---|---|---|
| B-6 | Helps the body make red blood cells, converts tryptophan to niacin, and contributes to immunity and nervous system function; used in metabolism of proteins and fats | Meats, fish, poultry, legumes, leafy green vegetables, potatoes, bananas, fortified cereals | 2 milligrams/day |
| Biotin | Contributes to energy production and metabolism of proteins, fats, and carbohydrates | Found in many foods, especially liver, egg yolks, cereal | 300 micrograms/day |
| B-12 | Important for proper nerve function; works with folate, converting it to an active form; helps make red blood cells and helps metabolize proteins and fats | Only found in animal foods, such as meats, fish, poultry, milk, cheese, eggs, or in fortified cereals. | 6 micrograms/day |

(Continued)

| WHAT | WHY | WHERE TO GET IT | RECOMMENDATION FOR MEN AGES 11 AND UP |
|------|-----|-----------------|----------------------------------------|
| Vitamin C | Important for immune function, acts as an antioxidant, strengthens blood vessels and capillary walls, makes collagen and connective tissue that hold muscles and bones together, helps form scar tissue, keeps gums healthy, and helps the body absorb iron from foods | Many fruits and vegetables, especially citrus fruits, dark green vegetables, strawberries, papaya, cantaloupe, peppers, broccoli, potatoes, tomatoes | 60 milligrams/day |
| Calcium | Critical for strengthening bones and teeth, proper nervous system and immune function, muscle contraction, blood clotting, and blood pressure | Dairy products, including milk, yogurt, and cheese, fish with bones (such as sardines or salmon), tofu, legumes, broccoli, kale, cabbage, calcium-fortified orange juice | 800 milligrams/day |

| WHAT | WHY | WHERE TO GET IT | RECOMMENDATION FOR MEN AGES 11 AND UP |
|------|-----|-----------------|-----------------------------------------|
| Chloride | Important for fluid balance in the body, and digestion, since it is a component of hydrochloric acid found in the stomach | Table salt, soy sauce, processed foods | 750 milligrams/day |
| Chromium | Works with insulin to help cells use glucose | Unrefined whole grain products, liver, brewer's yeast, nuts, cheese, meats | 50-200 micrograms/day |
| Copper | Helps make red blood cells, is part of several body enzymes, and is important for the absorption of iron | Shellfish, nuts, seeds, legumes, whole grain products, liver, meats | 1.5-3.0 milligrams/day |
| Vitamin D | Increases absorption of calcium and phosphorus, which leads to stronger bones and teeth | The body can make vitamin D on its own, provided it gets enough sunlight. By exposing face, hands, and forearms for between 5 and | |

*(Continued)*

| WHAT | WHY | WHERE TO GET IT | RECOMMENDATION FOR MEN AGES 11 AND UP |
|---|---|---|---|
| **Vitamin D** *(Continued)* | | 30 minutes two or three times per week, most people can manufacture all the vitamin D they need. Sunscreen blocks the type of rays needed to produce vitamin D. | 10 micrograms/day (equivalent to about 400 IU) |
| **Vitamin E** | Acts as an antioxidant, reducing risks of cancer and heart disease; contributes to good immunity | Vegetable oils, wheat germ, whole grain products, nuts, egg yolks, green leafy vegetables | 10 milligrams/day (equivalent to about 30 IU) |
| **Folate** (Folic Acid) | Critical for all cell functions, since folate helps make DNA and RNA; may protect against heart disease by lowering homocysteine levels | Leafy green vegetables, especially spinach and turnip greens, legumes, broccoli, asparagus, oranges, fortified cereals | 400 micrograms/day |

| WHAT | WHY | WHERE TO GET IT | RECOMMENDATION FOR MEN AGES 11 AND UP |
|---|---|---|---|
| Fluoride | Helps form bones and teeth; helps make teeth decay resistant | Fluoridated drinking water, seafood, tea | 1.5-2.5 milligrams/day |
| Iodine | Regulates growth and metabolic rate as a component of thyroid hormones | Iodized table salt, salt water fish | 150 micrograms/day |
| Iron | Important part of red blood cells | Red meat, fish, poultry, eggs, legumes, fortified cereals | 10 milligrams/day |
| Magnesium | Part of enzymes in the body, helps build bones, teeth, and proteins; important for proper function of nerves, muscles, and immune system | Legumes, nuts, whole grain foods, green vegetables, seafood | 420 milligrams/day |
| Manganese | Part of many body enzymes | Widely available in foods, especially nuts, leafy green vegetables, tea, unrefined cereals and grain products. | 2-5 milligrams/day |

*(Continued)*

| WHAT | WHY | WHERE TO GET IT | RECOMMENDATION FOR MEN AGES 11 AND UP |
|------|-----|-----------------|----------------------------------------|
| Phosphorus | Works with calcium to form bones and teeth, helps create energy in the body, is part of cell membranes; is present in DNA and RNA, the body's genetic material | Most prevalent in protein-rich foods, such as meat, poultry, fish, eggs, and milk | 700 milligrams/day |
| Potassium | Important for nerve transmission, muscle contraction, and balance of fluids in the body | Many types of fresh foods, including meat, milk, whole grain products, fruits, legumes, potatoes | 2000 milligrams/day |
| Selenium | Powerful antioxidant that works to protect cells from damage; important for cell growth | Seafood, meats, grain products, seeds | 70 micrograms/day |

| WHAT | WHY | WHERE TO GET IT | RECOMMENDATION FOR MEN AGES 11 AND UP |
|---|---|---|---|
| Zinc | Part of many enzymes in the body; helps with tissue growth and wound healing; important for taste perception | Protein-rich foods, including meat, poultry, fish | 15 milligrams/day |

As always, a caution. There is a dark side to dietary supplements. Supplements are not widely regulated. As with food, federal law requires manufacturers of dietary supplements to ensure that the products they put on the market are safe. So unless the supplement makers want the Feds on their ass, they're going to make their products safe. That doesn't mean they're going to make the products effective.

See, supplements are not drugs. If they were, they'd be regulated by the Food and Drug Administration. And the FDA defines drugs as things that are intended to diagnose, cure, mitigate, treat, or prevent diseases. Before marketing, drugs must undergo clinical studies to determine their effectiveness, safety, possible interactions with other substances, and appropriate dosages. The FDA must review these data and authorize the drugs' uses before they are marketed. If the drug successfully makes it through that process, its makers can claim that it "reduces butt swelling" or whatever. Dietary supplements can't make such specific claims because they haven't gone through the full FDA review.

That's not to say that there's no telling what's in a dietary supplement. There is. The Dietary Supplement Health and Education

Act (DSHEA), passed in 1994, sees to that. Traditionally, dietary supplements referred to products made of one or more of the essential nutrients, such as vitamins, minerals, and protein. But DSHEA broadened the definition to include, with some exceptions, any product intended for ingestion as a supplement to the diet. This includes vitamins; minerals; herbs, botanicals, and other plant-derived substances; and amino acids (the individual building blocks of protein) and concentrates, metabolites, constituents, and extracts of these substances. Most important, DSHEA requires manufacturers to include the words "dietary supplement" on their product labels. Also, a "supplement facts" panel is required on the labels of most dietary supplements. This way you know what the product you're buying is made from. And that's nice.

In summary, all adults can probably benefit from one multivitamin per day. For a few pennies per day, a multivitamin provides added insurance that adequate intake of the daily necessary vitamins and micronutrients will be met. However, supplements do not provide all the known—and perhaps unknown —nutritional benefits of conventional food. In other words, you still have to eat right.

## Water Boy

Although we have discussed dietary guidelines, the building blocks (carbs, proteins, and fats), and nutritional supplements, we have yet to discuss the most important supplement of all— WATER! Water makes up over 60 percent of your body's overall composition and is very important in many ways other than quenching your thirst (author's note: the clean, crisp, mountain water in Coors does not count as water). Studies have shown that aside from reducing the risk of kidney stones, bladder cancer, and heart attacks, water can:

- Flush out the body's toxins

- Lube up your joints

- Decrease exercised-induced asthma

- Increase your mental alertness (the brain is three-quarters water—dry it up to be dumb)

- Increase blood flow

- Increase erectile performance (that's water, not scotch and water)

Although water is important to your health, it becomes even more important when you drink coffee, tea, sodas, or alcohol or work out because you can become dehydrated. A simple rule of thumb is for every coffee, tea, soda, or glass of alcohol have two glasses of water. The *International Journal of Sports Medicine* suggests that you drink a glass of water every fifteen or twenty minutes during a workout (which equates to approximately 150 percent of the amount of sweat lost during a typical hour-long workout).

## Jumping on the Bandwagon

Although water is one of the keys to proper health, many savvy companies have started to market their wares under the veil of water. And, in doing this, many dads think they are "doing good" by drinking lots of water. But more calories are sneaking into their diets without even knowing it. Here's an example:

| Product | Calories |
| --- | --- |
| Aquafina Essentials | 100 |
| Gatorade Propel | 30 |
| Hanse's $E_2O$ | 120 |
| Snapple Elements | 100 |
| Vitaminwater (Glaceau) | 125 |

Bottled water also may not be better than good, old-fashioned tap water, despite its reputation among some for a "cleaner" taste. Bottled water frequently contains less than the recommended levels of fluoride, which could cause a rise in tooth decay among children. And bottled water is not as pure as many people think, according to a recent report.

Experts writing in the journal *Archives of Family Medicine* say the same standards should apply to both tap and bottled water, because bottled water is more and more often used as a substitute for tap water. For the study, researchers took tap water samples from four processing plants in Cleveland and compared them with five types of bottled water samples, measuring fluoride and bacteria levels in both. Only 5 percent of the bottled water purchased in Cleveland fell within the fluoride range recommended by the state, and nearly 90 percent of the bottled water samples contained less than a third of the fluoride recommended.

Not only did 100 percent of the tap water samples fall within the recommended range, but all of it was within 0.04 percent of hitting the state's *optimal* fluoride-level mark—1.0 mg of fluoride per liter. And while two-thirds of the bottled water samples did indeed have a lower bacterial count than the tap water samples, 25 percent had a whopping ten times more bacteria. Bacteria in tap water samples varied only slightly.

Even though the EPA recently required that local water systems regularly report the quality of the local tap water to the community, no similar proposals requiring bottled water to report its quality on its label are on the table, researchers note.

So for all of you dads that are trying to be water snobs like the other country club gents—just go for the tap. No—not the beer kind.

### PLAYBOOK NOTES: Now a Word from Our Supplement Sponsor

1. Most dads don't eat a well-balanced diet, so they may want to take supplements.

2. The supplement industry is not regulated, so buy your vitamins from a reputable source.

3. Drink plenty of water! Due to the fluoride content, tap water may be your best bet.

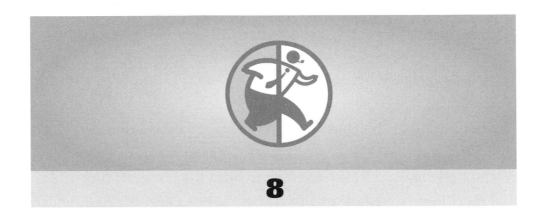

**8**

# Fitness—The Framework

"No one ever drowned in sweat."
—LOU HOLTZ

Okay, men, take a knee and listen up. We're going to go over the core philosophy for the Fat Daddy program. This is going to get you and keep you in shape, and there's no time to lollygag around. Let's get to it.

This chapter will be arranged like so:

- **Quitters never win, and winners never quit:** How to get over procrastination and score points in four down territory.

- **Proper play calling:** Gym lingo and etiquette and other basics.

- **The Fat Daddy Four Quarters Workout:** stretching, aerobic activity, weight training, and yoga.

- **Cover the middle:** Simple exercises to get back those abs of steel.

■ **Away games:** Tips for exercising while on the road, at the office, or in the car.

■ **Extra points:** How exercise can improve your sex life.

Before we go any further, you must recognize how important exercise is to being considered "healthy." Over the past two decades, researchers have been pouring over treadmill data, mortality tables, and nutritional pyramids to answer two basic questions. First, which or what exercises correlate to longer life in men? Second, which fitness programs tackle debilitating diseases like arthritis and diabetes most effectively?

You're probably familiar with *aerobic* workouts. But did you know the word means "with air"? Yeah, I didn't think so. Aerobic activity is your body's ability to supply fresh oxygen-rich blood to your muscles and organs (and therefore defining your level of *endurance*). It's key to good fitness.

But so is *strength*. Researchers at the Honolulu Heart Project studied a group of men for twenty years and found the strongest (measured by a mechanical grip tester) had a two to three times better chance of being free of chronic illnesses as they got older.

So strong is good, and aerobics are good. But here's the rub. Even if you improve your strength, boost your endurance, and do aerobics regularly, you're still getting older. And probably balder. And you may be getting less of something else. But you're going to have to talk to your wives and girlfriends about that. I can't help you there. Point being: As you age, tendons, ligaments, and muscles become more brittle and rigid. You can fight this, though. For the hair, there's Rogaine. For the rest of the body, there's stretching. See, unlike women, most men's muscle and ligament fibers are naturally tight. That's why many women can do a split with little effort while when most men do a split they scream bloody murder. But with a long-term commitment to regular stretching, that can change. Over time, if you stretch regularly men can promote permanent gains in flexibility by stretching. And you're never too old to start.

My father is a good example. "Wild Bill," as his friends call him (only because he's anything but) started a morning stretching ritual fifty years ago to help him with an aching lower back. Today he still religiously does a series of stretches each morning while still wearing his musty, silk pj's. Honestly, it's a gruesome sight. And I'm pretty sure that witnessing it has scarred me for life. But it has made the old man one of the most flexible and fit eighty-two-year-olds you'll ever meet.

This, when you think about it, is really not that surprising. A recent article in the *Journal of the American Medical Association* reported that a study of 45,000 men showed exercise increased heart health. Men who ran for at least an hour each week had a 42 percent reduced risk for developing heart disease and dying. Lifting weights for thirty minutes or more per week cut the risk 23 percent, while rowing an hour or more per week cut the risk by about 18 percent. Even walking briskly each day for at least thirty minutes led to an 18 percent reduction in heart disease risk. And the faster the men walked the more benefit they gained—regardless of how long they walked. These protective effects of exercise were seen in all ages and in men who were overweight or had a family history of heart disease.

In other words, just like I said, it is never too late to start, and the sooner you get started, the better chance you'll have of passing on good health habits to your own kids. Wild Bill is living proof of that. But, really, do your kids a favor and trade the pj's for sweats. Or at least close the door.

## Quitters Never Win, and Winners Never Quit

Dads have to cram more into a day than ever before. It's like a two-minute drill—you've got a long way to go in a very short amount of time, and you *have* to score. But the Fat Daddy Game Plan will get you into the end zone. The key to success is planning. Let's say you work out at night and your wife says to you, in that loving voice of hers, "I would much rather you work out in the morning because that will give you more time with the family in the evening." Or, more realistically, let's say she says, "Hey, Dr. Exercise, if you ever want some again, you'd better get out of the gym and start giving me a hand around the house at night." Of course, she wins. So just do it. If you have to get up at 6 A.M. instead of 7 A.M. to catch a brisk walk and some stretching, so be it. Remember, all you need is a cumulative sixty minutes per day. If you can schedule a lunch date or have time to sit in traffic, you've got time for exercise. This is key: Your daily exercise is just like a football team's daily practice. They don't miss practice, you can't miss your workout if you're going to win.

Here's something that works for me. I treat my daily exercise as a meeting. I block the time off in my organizer. I let my assistant know that workout time is part of my schedule, too. So, whether I'm going to the gym at 6 A.M. or noon or after hours, she knows not to schedule me with anything else for me at those times. This makes it a priority for me. And, if I have to miss a workout appointment, then I make sure I reschedule it just like I would any other important meeting.

If you follow that approach, you might also consider making your workout an appointment for two. You know what they say, "Couples that play together, stay together." No, really, they say that. A recent study at the University of Indiana found couples who worked out together stayed together 93.7 percent of the time. Conversely, those who worked out alone had 43 percent chance of a breakup. That alone should get you and your spouse sprinting together. And, come to think of it, this might explain some things. Mrs. Right and I never worked out together.

To be sure, no matter if you're working out with your wife or scheduling time in your organizer, or however you're making the commitment to regular workouts, everyone has "those days" when they don't seem to have the time or don't feel like exercising. But getting into any exercise groove requires a sense of motivation and determination—and you're the only one who can make yourself get off your ass. So get up and get off it before it gets any bigger.

Now, here are some simple plays to help you score when you have decided to commit to an exercise program:

- **First Down:** Register some forward progress. Commit to getting back in shape. That's your first play.

- **Second Down:** Keep moving the ball. Decide on specific goals. What do you want to look like? How soon can you get there? Are there any impending events that can provide extra motivation (like a class reunion) coming up? How are you going to measure your progress?

- **Third Down:** The big play. Design your workout routine based on your first and second down goal setting. Will you do weights or cardio, or hopefully both? How often? Where? With whom? Are you going to wear shorts or sweats? Are you going to listen to music to get you fired up? What about yoga? Can you take your family with you?

- **Fourth Down:** Last play to convert. Write down your goals and plans from the first three downs, get started, and stick with it. You can add or subtract what you like as your fitness level evolves. But above all, make sure you measure your progress. You can't manage what you can't measure.

Other tips that sometimes can help you get your workout juices flowing include everything from esoteric stuff like visualization and meditation to more tangible strategies like listening to inspirational music (I prefer Kiss, Metallica, or Linkin Park) or going to see an inspirational flick like *Remember the Titans* or *Rudy*.

## Proper Play Calling

There you are, dressed in all the right lycra and suddenly someone starts talking about abs, sets, and core. Ex-squeeze me? Baking powder? As if all the confusing information you sort through about exercise—how hard, how much, how often—isn't bad enough, consider the insider lingo you also have to get the hang of.

For some Fat Daddies (probably the Ex-Athlete Fat Daddy), exercise lingo is pretty well understood. Don't be too embarrassed if you don't talk the talk, though, because even some exercise enthusiasts don't have the jargon down. So before we start to talk about exercises, let's review some simple terminology so you won't come back to the huddle not knowing the plays.

| TERM | MEANING |
| --- | --- |
| Abs | Short for abdominal muscles. The muscular wall between your stomach and fat belly. |
| Aerobic | Means "with air." Aerobic activity is your body's ability to supply fresh oxygen-rich blood to your muscles and organs. Walking, running, swimming, biking, or anything that gets your heart rate up for at least twenty minutes are all "with air" exercises. |
| Anaerobic | Without air. Exercises include weight lifting, core training, some forms of yoga, and isometrics. |
| Barbell | The long weight bars that you hold with both hands, like when doing bench press. |

| TERM | MEANING |
| --- | --- |
| **Burn** | As in, "feeling the burn." No, you won't melt. This feeling usually comes at the end of a set when your muscles are exhausted and they begin to fatigue. |
| **Cardio** | Any form of aerobic activity. |
| **Core** | Core training is a relative new way of combining flexibility, agility, balancing, and strength training without using weights. Your core consists of the rectus abdominus, internal and external obliques, and erector spinaes, all the muscles in your midsection that allow you to transfer movement and power from the upper body to lower body and vice versa. |
| **Cut** (ripped or shredded) | Refers to a person with low body fat and a clearly defined and impressive muscle structure. (The Calvin Klein man is ripped.) |
| **Dumbbell** | The individual weight bars that are short enough to hold one in each hand. |
| **Form** | Correctly performing an exercise. |
| **Heart Rate** (maximum) | The fastest and hardest your heart muscle can theoretically beat (contract). Your personal redline. Maximum heart rates drop slowly with age, but not as fast or as much if you are fit. The standard formula for a proper maximum rate is 220 minus your age for men; error is 10-15 beats either way since heart rate maximums are genetically determined. |
| **Overtraining** | Doing so much exercise over time that your body can't recover. You feel weak, tired, and sore, but you don't want to stop working out. Sex, to the best of our knowledge, can't be overtrained. |

*(Continued)*

| TERM | MEANING |
|------|---------|
| Pump | Your muscles fill with blood and feel tight and firm. Then you're "pumped." This means you're attacking the right muscle fibers. It's a good feeling. |
| Range of Motion | The complete path of motion of an exercise. From the starting point to the muscle contraction and back to the starting point. New research has shown, however, that a partial range of motion (continuous arch) is safer and just as effective. |
| Reps | Short for "repetitions," this is how many times you will repeat an exercise in succession. |
| Sets/ Super Sets | A set is a consecutive grouping of "reps." A super set is two sets of different exercises that are done back-to-back consecutively without a rest. |
| Six Pack | What your abs look like when there is not a layer of blubber covering them. |
| Spotting | Ask your wife about this one, and watch her facial expression. But in the gym spotting means to stand by while someone lifts a weight as a safeguard in case the lifter needs assistance. If someone asks you to "spot" them, simply stand ready while they are lifting, but don't touch the bar or weight he or she is using. Just be alert. Once the person's lifting rhythm slows, lightly use your fingers or hands to help maintain the pace. Don't suddenly grab or lift the weight for the person, but don't wait too long either. |
| Stretching | Lengthening of muscles and soft tissues by reaching to the point where you must stop and holding. Safest method is static; most unsafe is ballistic (where you bounce your body weight into a stretch). |

| TERM | MEANING |
|---|---|
| **Strip** | Did you know that Dallas has more strip bars per capita than any other city in the nation? But I digress. The term "to strip," in the weight room, means to take the weight plates off the ends of the bars or from the machines and to return them to their proper racks (or "to rack them"). Sort of like putting away your toys when you're done. The same cleaning-up applies when you use dumbbells, the small weights you hold in each hand. They should be returned to their racks and not left lying on the floor. |
| **Warm Up** | Light activity to be done for at least ten minutes before any exercise is attempted (walking, stretching, stationary bike, etc.). |
| **"Working In"** | To "work in" means to alternate with someone else on one piece of equipment. If you're using a machine and someone poses that question, then bustles onto your bench, don't be intimidated and leave. They're asking politely to use the equipment with you. Just step aside, let the person do the exercise, step back for your turn, and alternate quickly until done. Don't be afraid to ask that question if you need a particular machine that's occupied. Just wait until the person is taking a break and, like a weight-lifting pro, pop the question: "Can I work in?" |

Now that you have the proper lingo, let's talk about workout etiquette. Health clubs, country clubs, or just plain old gyms are social gathering places just like malls, coffee shops, and workplaces. Even if you're partly or fully naked some of the time—or maybe especially because of that—basic rules of group politeness apply. Here are a few simple guidelines to follow.

- **Throw in the towel.** You don't want to sit in someone else's sweat. Don't make them sit in yours. After using any type of exercise equipment, be sure to wipe it off. Covering the seats or benches with a towel beforehand helps to avoid this problem, and it also protects you from germs that can be passed on through other people's sweat.

- **Share your toys.** If you are lifting weights, trade sets with someone else. This way you can rest while someone else lifts. Cardio equipment needs to be shared as well. Many clubs have time limits for these machines during peak hours.

- **Don't be cheesy.** My college roommate never washed his biking shorts after working out. By senior year they could bike all by themselves. Don't be that way. Wash your workout clothes on a regular basis. Also, leave the Hi Karate at home. It reeks.

- **Don't be a turn on.** If you turn on your phone at the gym, someone may slap you with a dumbbell. Turn it off. Concentrate.

- **Clean up.** If you like to read while on an exercise bike, make sure to properly dispose of newspapers and magazines when you're done. Recycling is nice, but trash is acceptable, too. Or you might consider offering your materials to others, especially if the materials contain pictures of half-naked women.

## The Fat Daddy Four Quarters Workout

Now that you know the lingo and how not to behave like a schlub, let's look at the *Fat Daddy Four Quarters Workout*.

This is no ordinary exercise program. The Fat Daddy plan is a wholesale lifestyle change that's easy to use, easy to implement, and easy to stick with. So there.

The program consists of four fitness disciplines (or quarters) composed of stretching, aerobic activity, weight training, and yoga. You simply pick two disciplines per day, do four exercise per discipline, and alternate disciplines over the week. You will end up working out four times a week while gaining strength, flexibility and cardiovascular endurance. One exception. Abs should be done every other day.

## First Quarter: Stretching

- **Time:** Morning and after a workout

- **Frequency:** Four times per week

- **Routine:** Pick four stretches (two upper body, two lower body)

- **Benefit:** Increases flexibility and prevents injury

## Second Quarter: Aerobic Activity (Cardio)

- **Time:** Best in the morning

- **Frequency:** Four times per week

- **Routine:** Pick a different exercise each time (see Sample Week table)

- **Benefit:** Improves function of the heart and lungs and burns fat

## Third Quarter: Weight Training

■ **Time:** Best in the afternoon

■ **Frequency:** Four times per week

■ **Routine:** One body part per day (See Sample Week table)

■ **Benefit:** Tones and shapes muscles, speeds metabolism, and strengthens bones

## Fourth Quarter: Yoga

■ **Time:** Anytime

■ **Frequency:** Four times per week

■ **Routine:** A minimum of four poses per workout

■ **Benefit:** Increases flexibility, circulation, and strength and helps build a stronger immune system

| SAMPLE WEEK | | | | | | | |
|---|---|---|---|---|---|---|---|
| QUARTER | MON. | TUES. | WED. | THURS. | FRI. | SAT. | SUN. |
| Stretching | X | | X | | | X | X |
| Cardio | X | | | X | X | | X |
| Weights | | X | X | X | | X | |
| Yoga | | X | | X | X | X | |
| Abs | X | | X | | X | | X |

# Stretching

Many gurus and experts talk about the benefits of proper diet, cardiovascular activity, and weight training, but there are also many overlooked health benefits in the simple act of stretching. These range from filling the muscles with oxygen-rich blood and nourishing joints to relieving tension and preventing fitness-related injuries. Stretching doesn't mean doing the splits. What we're talking about is functional stretching—stretching for mobility and flexibility in everyday tasks, like twisting maneuvers while grabbing the seat belt or reaching for a beer. You should try to stretch every day, preferably a nice, easy stretch in the morning—you can even do this in bed (insert your own joke there)—or a slow stretch before a workout, and a deeper, longer stretch after you work out. Fifteen minutes, tops, in any of those cases.

Here are a couple points to remember.

- **Before and after.** Try to do some light stretching before you work out, and longer, deeper stretches after you work out. Aside from all the physical benefits, stretching after a workout will help you cool down and relax. And while we're on the subject of warming up and cooling down, also note that you should do some light walking, take a warm shower or bath, or ride a bike for at least five minutes before you do any type of stretching.

- **No-pain-no-gain is bad.** Stretching is supposed to be relaxing and should not be painful. If you reach your pain point, back off.

- **Don't go ballistic.** Ballistic stretching is bouncing while you stretch. You probably used to do this is gym glass. Turns out your gym teacher was a moron. Basically, it's bouncing when you stretch that is bad. Bouncing while stretching risks tearing muscles and tendons. Bad idea.

- **Do a big-word stretch.** One type of stretching is called proprioceptive neuromuscular facilitation, but there's no point in remembering that. Remember it as PNF if you must, or just know that this type of stretching is excellent. Basically PNF is where you stretch out to a certain point, then contract or "flex" at that point, then relax for a moment and continue the stretch even farther.

■ **Hold the static.** Static stretching is generally the way to go. Gently go into a stretch until you feel the resistance in the muscle. Then hold that position for thirty seconds while taking full deep breaths.

Have you ever seen a stressed-out cat? Me neither. And I'm convinced that besides the whole all-you-can-eat, sleep-all-day lifestyle, part of a cat's nonchalance has to do with stretching. Cats stretch all the time. Fitness instructors will even tell their clients to do a "cat stretch" to emulate the things. I'm probably a bit more selective than a cat when I stretch, but I think I come out just as relaxed. My stretching time is a moment of peace. I relax, think about my day, my workout, my kids, or nothing at all. It's a great way to start the day, and the only way to end a workout.

Here are some of the best stretches you can add to your workout. *Pick four stretches per workout.*

(two upper body, and two lower body)

| STRETCH | UPPER BODY | LOWER BODY |
|---|---|---|
| Lower Back | | X |
| Quadriceps | | X |
| Hamstring | | X |
| Calf | | X |
| Pretzel | X | X |
| Upper Back | X | |
| Chest | X | |
| Shoulder | X | |

## Lower Back Stretch

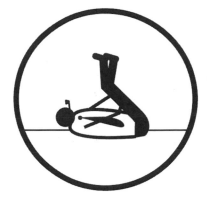

1. **Muscles Stretched:** Lower back and butt.
2. **Starting Point:** Lie flat on your back.
3. **The Move:** Gently raise both of your knees to your chest, as if you're trying to roll yourself into a ball. Focus on pressing you lower back against the floor and breathe normally. Hold for thirty seconds and gently release this "tucked" position.
4. **Tip:** Take big, deep breaths.

## Quadriceps Stretch

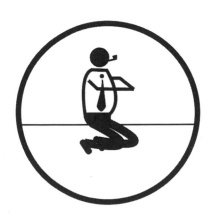

1. **Muscles Worked:** Front of your upper leg (quadriceps).
2. **Starting Point:** Gently sit on your heels with your knees parallel to each other.
3. **The Move:** Slowly sit farther back onto your heels while keeping your back tight and torso erect. Hold for thirty seconds; repeat.
4. **Tip:** Place your arms in front of you for balance.

### Hamstring Stretch

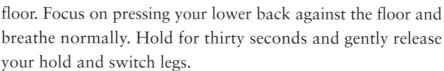

1. **Muscles Stretched:** Back of legs (hamstrings).
2. **Starting Point:** Lie flat on your back.
3. **The Move:** Grab the back of one leg and gently raise it perpendicular to your body. Keep your other leg and back flat on the floor. Focus on pressing your lower back against the floor and breathe normally. Hold for thirty seconds and gently release your hold and switch legs.
4. **Tip:** Slightly raise your chin to help keep your back pressed to the floor.

### Calf Stretch

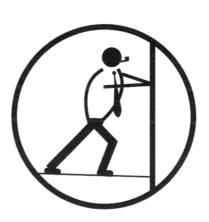

1. **Muscles Stretched:** Calves and Achilles tendon.
2. **Starting Point:** Standing.
3. **The Move:** Leaning against a wall with your arms extended, bend one leg at the knee while keeping the other leg behind you straight. Feel the stretch in your calf on the leg that is extended. Stretch until you feel a concentrated "burn" in your calf. Hold twenty seconds and release. Switch legs and repeat.
4. **Tip:** Keep your extended knee straight.

## Pretzel Stretch

1. **Muscles Stretched:** Lower back and butt.
2. **Starting Point:** Lie flat on your back with your knees bent and feet flat.
3. **The Move:** Cross your left ankle over your right upper thigh by your knee. Tighten your abdominals as you bring your right knee toward your chest until you feel a stretch in the right buttock. Hold twenty seconds, repeat, and switch legs.
4. **Tip:** Keep your shoulders and back flat on the floor, and remember to breathe.

## Upper Back Stretch

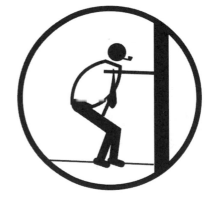

1. **Muscles Worked:** Upper back.
2. **Starting Point:** Standing.
3. **Tho Movo:** Start by finding a stationary object that can support your weight. While standing, bend at the waist and grab the object (with your arm straight), twisting your wrist and facing your palm out. Hold the stationary object and lean back. Gently try to rotate your hips out away from the arm that is extended. You should be able to feel a strong pull in the outer portion of you back. That's good. It means you're hitting the right spot. Hold for twenty seconds, breathe normally, repeat, and switch sides.
4. **Tip.** Go very slow; rotate your hips away from the stretch.

## Chest Stretch

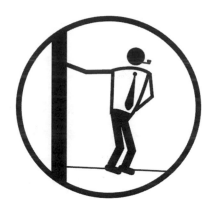

1. **Muscles Stretched:** Chest, biceps, shoulders.
2. **Starting Point:** Standing.
3. **The Move:** Standing straight with your knees slightly bent, take one arm and brace it against a stationary object (a wall, tree, door jamb). Your arm should be extended to chest level. Slightly bend the extended arm at the elbow, and rotate the rest of your body slightly in the opposite direction. You should feel the stretch in your chest. Hold twenty seconds, repeat, and switch to the other side.
4. **Tip.** Your (stretching side) elbow should be parallel with your shoulder.

## Shoulder Stretch

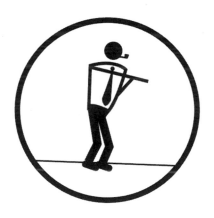

1. **Muscles Stretched:** Shoulders.
2. **Starting Point:** Standing.
3. **The Move:** Stand straight, stomach in, shoulders square to your body. Take one arm and cross it across your body parallel with your shoulders. Support the arm at the elbow with the opposite arm. You should feel the stretch in the shoulder area in the arm that you are crossing across your body. Hold stretch twenty seconds, repeat, and switch sides.
4. **Tip:** Keep stretched arm parallel to your body.

# Aerobic (Cardio) Activity

If you are going to be fit, you have to do cardio. Yes. You have to. Stop whining. As we discussed earlier, cardiovascular/aerobic activity is your body's ability to supply fresh oxygen-rich blood to your muscles and organs. It defines your level of endurance, and, more important, doing it can save your life.

The goal of cardio exercise is to keep your heart rate at 60 percent to 80 percent of your maximum heart rate for at least forty minutes. (The attorneys insist I offer a warning here, so please consult with your physician prior to starting any exercise program. Of course, you already knew that.) Your target maximum heart rate is the theoretical maximum number of beats per minute your heart can pulse without breaking down. That's roughly 220 beats per minute for men and 226 for women. The heart muscle can take a little less as we get older. So you subtract your age from 220. That's your personal maximum heart rate.

By "maximum," I mean, "not where you really want to be during a workout." For a moderate aerobic workout, experts recommend sticking to a pulse between 60 and 80 percent of your maximum. So a thirty-five-year-old man (220 – 35 = 185 maximum) should exercise with a pulse between 111 and 148 beats per minute. (185 × .60 = 111. 185 × .80 = 180. Math = fun.) Novice exercisers should stick to the lower end of the range.

By the way, the resting heart rate for most individuals is around 60 to 85 beats per minute. But people in top condition and high endurance athletes have a resting heart rate that's usually just 35 to 55 beats per minute. Those lucky bastards.

To check your own heart rate. Get a watch and count how many beats you feel over sixty seconds when you do one of the following:

- Press your index and middle finger to one side of your neck, locating a big-ass vein (or, as "doctors" call it, the carotid artery).

- Press your palm over the left side of the chest (where, "doctors" say you can find your "heart").

- Press your index and middle finger between the base of your thumb and your wrist where there's a smaller-ass vein that those same "doctors" call your radial artery (between the base of your thumb and your wrist).

Now that you know where your pulse should be and how to track it, try to check it as you do your cardio workouts. The longer you stay in your target heart rate zone, the more fat you'll burn.

I've offered a list below of aerobic activities. Choose any. Choose all. But whichever you pick, do the exercise *four* times per week for at least forty minutes each time. If you can't go forty minutes at a speedy clip, just slow down, but try to keep going. You'll work your way up. And if the exercise bores you, then bring your wife or kids or a friend with you, listen to music, something. Just don't give yourself an excuse for not getting out there.

A word of caution, though. If you're in a major city, try to avoid outdoor aerobics between 5 P.M. and 7 P.M. The air sucks worse than the traffic in the evening rush hour. And the carbon monoxide you'll inhale will more than outweigh the health benefits of the workout. It's kind of like shooting hoops while smoking a stogie—dumb.

## SAMPLE "FAT MELTING" CARDIO EXERCISES

| ACTIVITY | CALORIES BURNED (40 MIN) | TOTAL WEIGHT LOST AFTER 8 WEEKS @ 4X PER WEEK |
|---|---|---|
| Running (8 min. mile) | 656 | 4.5 lbs. |
| Jumping rope | 524 | 3.6 lbs. |
| Stair climbing | 540 | 3.7 lbs. |
| Basketball | 472 | 3.2 lbs. |
| Tennis | 460 | 3.2 lbs. |
| Cycling (14 mph) | 440 | 3.0 lbs. |
| Swimming | 408 | 2.8 lbs. |
| Walking (4 mph) | 312 | 2.1 lbs. |
| Golf | 272 | 1.9 lbs. |

*\* based upon a 175-pound dad.*

## Weight (Resistance) Training

Outside of water, muscle makes up the majority of our body. Every part of our body is affected by muscles. Smiling requires muscles. So do bowel movements—sorry, it's true. And, yes, you're also using muscles in the bedroom. Hopefully regularly. And hopefully with someone else.

Because muscles make up so much of our bodies, keeping them strong and fit can affect our minds. Weight training can play an important role in the development of self-confidence. Think about it. Weight training will increase strength, build and tone muscles, and increase muscular endurance. In other words,

### TRICK PLAY

A great way to tighten up your midsection is to contract your abdominal muscles while carrying out your cardiovascular routine. Whether you're running or stair climbing, focus on contracting your ab muscles in the last three or four minutes of each cardiovascular workout.

you'll feel stronger. That'll make you feel tougher, more rugged, more like a man.

Weight training can also help you maintain lean body mass. That's important for individuals attempting weight loss, but it also decreases the risk of osteoporosis, develops coordination and balance, and prevents injuries resulting from weak muscles. You might not notice some of that, but you will notice your pants fitting better and your biceps pushing out from under shirtsleeves more. And that development has a huge impact on how you feel about yourself.

Something else is important here. Studies have shown that most men lose about 30 percent of their muscle mass between the ages of twenty and seventy. Much of that loss occurs because of inactivity. But it is not inevitable. In "sedentary" muscles, cells shrink and become weaker. So weight training will help you slow down this aging process. And how often do you get to reverse the signs of aging without Viagra?

There are other advantages to weight training, of course. So, herewith the **Fat Daddy Top Twenty** reasons to hit the iron. Weight training:

1. Increases your resting basal metabolism—that's fitness speak—which causes you to burn more calories. You'll even burn more calories while you're sleeping.

2. Makes you stronger.

3. Has a positive affect on almost all of your 650-plus muscles.

4. Increases your blood's level of HDL cholesterol (the good type).

5. Builds stronger muscles, stabilizes joints and connective tissues.

6. Improves posture.

7. Builds endurance for daily activities (e.g., traveling, lifting groceries, lifting children, or mowing the lawn).

8. Makes you less prone to lower-back injuries.

9. Improves your balance and coordination.

10. Improves your mood.

11. Decreases resting blood pressure.

12. Decreases your risk of developing adult onset diabetes.

13. Decreases anxiety.

14. Lowers your resting heart rate, a sign of a more efficient heart.

15. Stimulates bone growth, which helps retard osteoporosis.

16. Improves the functioning of your immune system.

17. Gives you a leaner, *sexier* physique.

18. Makes your clothes fit better.

19. Makes you more attractive to the opposite sex.

20. See 17-19 and guess what else can result from weight training. Oh, yes.

Over the past twenty years, I have competed in many different sports from boxing and bodybuilding to football and power-lifting. I have been exposed to hundreds of different types of weight training exercises from some of the most knowledgeable coaches and trainers around. That's a lot of time spent in the company of hairy, sweaty men, and, let's face it, not everything I've seen was a pretty sight. But it was a small sacrifice for what I've learned. I now have a very unique perspective to what exercises work, how long they take to have an impact, and what the proper training techniques are. In the rest of this section, I have tried to boil that knowledge down to simple groups of exercises that any Fat Daddy can follow.

But let's be honest. As in everything worth doing, weight training requires a great deal of effort and a lot patience to see results. There's no magic muscle belt that'll get you there while you eat nachos and watch bowling on TV. You've got to make the effort. No, you probably won't end up having to shower with as many men as I have, but you will have to sacrifice time and you will have to make a concerted effort. Trust me, though, the payoff will be worth your investment.

## FAT DADDY WEIGHT TRAINING METHODOLOGY

| WEEK 1 | WEEK 2 | WEEK 3 | REPEAT WEEK 1 AND INCREASE THE WEIGHT AS MUCH AS POSSIBLE WHILE ACHIEVING THE SAME NUMBER OF REPS/REP RATIO |
|---|---|---|---|
| Light weight | Medium weight | Heavy weight | Light weight |
| One set | Two sets | Three sets | One set |
| 20 reps | 20 reps | 12 reps | 20 reps |
| 40 second rest between exercises | 40 second rest between exercises | Two minute rest between exercises | 40 second rest between exercises |

Pick *three exercises* and *two body parts* to exercise per workout. Abs, as I mentioned before, should be done every other day. Also, exercise your largest muscle groups first and descend your exercises to the smallest muscle group. The reason behind this is simple. If you fatigue the smaller muscle groups first, you won't have enough strength to use the bigger muscles fully.

| CHEST | SHOULDERS | BACK | ARMS- *BICEPS* | ARMS- *TRICEPS* | LEGS | ABS |
|-------|-----------|------|----------------|-----------------|------|-----|
| Bench press | Shoulder press | Chin-ups | Seated barbell curls (preacher style) | Press downs | Squats | Crunches |
| Incline press | Side laterals | Pull downs | Dumbbell curls | French press | Lunges | Reverse crunches/ Leg raises |
| Dips | Bent over laterals | Cable rows | Concentration curls | Kickbacks | Curls or stiff leg dead lifts | Cable crunches |
| Cable crossovers | Cable laterals | Hyper-extensions | Cable curls | Overhead extensions | Extensions | Toe touches |
| Dips | Shrugs | One-arm rows | | | Lunges | Plank |

## Bench Press

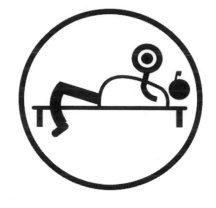

1. **Primary Muscles Worked:** Chest.
2. **Secondary Muscles Worked:** Shoulders, triceps.
3. **The Move:** Lying flat on a bench, grasp the bar and lower to your chest. Once at your chest, press up to the starting position.
4. **Tip:** When lowering the weight inhale, when pressing the weight exhale. Remember to keep your feet flat on the floor and buttocks flat on the bench.

## Incline Press

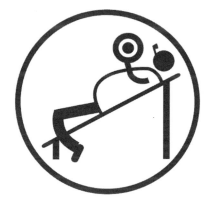

1. **Primary Muscles Worked:** Chest.
2. **Secondary Muscles Worked:** Shoulders.
3. **The Move:** Using a barbell or dumbbell, lie on a 45-degree angle bench. Lower the weight to your upper chest just below your neck. Elbows should be out to your side. Push the weight back to the starting position (with a slight arch) while almost locking out your elbows. Repeat.
4. **Tip:** Your elbows should be slightly bent, and the motion should resemble hugging a barrel.

### Cable Crossovers

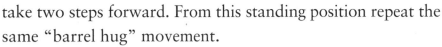

1. **Primary Muscles Worked:** Chest.
2. **Secondary Muscles Worked:** Shoulders.
3. **The Move:** Standing between a dual cable machine, grasp the cable handles that are in the upper setting. While holding the cable handles in each hand, take two steps forward. From this standing position repeat the same "barrel hug" movement.
4. **Tip:** Keep elbows slightly bent at all times, and try to do the movement slowly.

### Reverse Dips

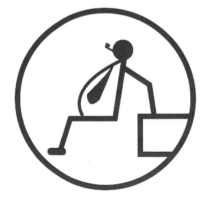

1. **Primary Muscles Worked:** Chest.
2. **Secondary Muscles Worked:** Shoulders, triceps.
3. **The Move:** Sit on the edge of a bench, stool, ledge, chair, or rock. Sit on your hands and slowly slide your feet forward and your butt off a chair or something about 24 inches off the ground. "Dip" down as low as you can go with your bum toward the ground. Then press back up to the starting position. Repeat.
4. **Tip:** For added help, don't go as deep, and keep you feet closer to you.

### Shoulder Press

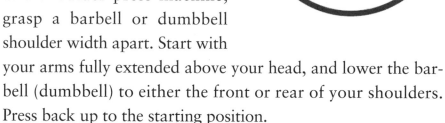

1. **Primary Muscles Worked:** Shoulders.
2. **Secondary Muscles Worked:** Triceps.
3. **The Move:** Sitting on a bench or at a shoulder press machine, grasp a barbell or dumbbell shoulder width apart. Start with your arms fully extended above your head, and lower the barbell (dumbbell) to either the front or rear of your shoulders. Press back up to the starting position.
4. **Tip:** Pressing to the front works the front of your shoulders (deltoids), pressing behind isolates the rear deltoids.

### Side Laterals

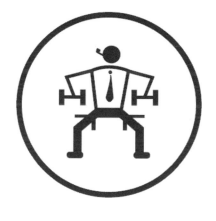

1. **Primary Muscles Worked:** Shoulders.
2. **Secondary Muscles Worked:** Trapezius.
3. **The Move:** Standing or sitting, take a pair of dumbbells and hold them at your sides. Raise your elbows and arms upward while turning your wrist as if you are pouring a pitcher of water. At the end position, your elbows should be at a 90-degree angle to your body.
4. **Tip:** If standing, bend your knees slightly. If sitting bend at the waist slightly. This exercise is properly done with lighter weight.

## Bent Over Laterals

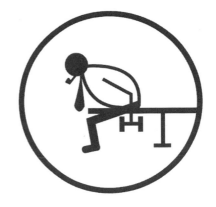

1. **Primary Muscles Worked:** Back of shoulders (rear deltoid).
2. **Secondary Muscles Worked:** Shoulders.
3. **The Move:** Sit on the end of a bench with your feet flat on the floor. Rest your chest almost to your knees. Grasp a dumb-bell in each hand. Raise your elbows behind you with your arms slightly bent. Feel the contraction in the rear part of your shoulders. Return weight to the starting position at your ankles.
4. **Tip:** In the up position slightly tilt your wrist like you are pour-ing a jug of milk. It will better isolate the muscle and take some pressure off your wrist.

## Side Laterals—Cable

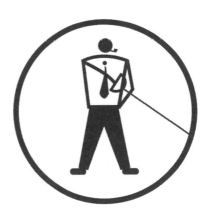

1. **Primary Muscles Worked:** Medial head or middle of the shoulder.
2. **Secondary Muscles Worked:** Trapezius.
3. **The Move:** Standing at a cable machine, reaching across your body grasp the cable handle that is in the lower position. Repeat the same motion as a dumbbell lateral using the cable while pulling across your body.
4. **Tip:** Use a light weight and do not swing.

## Shoulder Shrugs

1. **Primary Muscles Worked:** Trapezius.
2. **Secondary Muscles Worked:** Shoulders.
3. **The Move:** Standing or sitting grasp a barbell or dumbbell while your hands are positioned to your sides. Raise your shoulders as if you were shrugging "I don't know." Hold in the shrug position three seconds and relax.
4. **Tip:** None, it's idiot proof.

## Chin-Ups

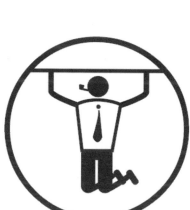

1. **Primary Muscles Worked:** Back (Latissimus Dorsi).
2. **Secondary Muscles Worked:** Biceps, shoulders.
3. **The Move:** These may be done raising your body to your chin or the back of your neck (this is referred to as a front or rear chin-up). Start in a hanging position. Pull your body up to the bar. That's it.
4. **Tip:** Do NOT swing.

## Pull Downs

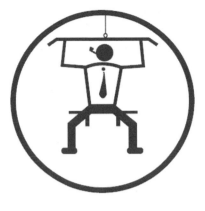

1. **Primary Muscles Worked:** Back (Latissimus Dorsi).
2. **Secondary Muscles Worked:** Biceps, shoulders.
3. **The Move:** While sitting on a lat pull machine, grasp the bar using a wide grip or a narrow grip. Pull the bar down to the top of the chest or the back of the neck.
4. **Tip:** As you are pulling the weight down, lean back slightly and gently arch your back. This helps isolate the movement and preserves your form. Again, do NOT swing.

## Hyperextensions

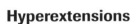

1. **Primary Muscles Worked:** Lower Back (Erector Spinae).
2. **Secondary Muscles Worked:** Glutes (butt), hamstrings, middle back.
3. **The Move:** Lying on a hyperextension machine, tuck your feet under the pad and cross your arms in front of your chest. Bend 45 degrees while keeping your back flat and raise yourself back to the starting extended position.
4. **Tip:** Go slow! If it hurts, STOP!

## Cable Rows

1. **Primary Muscles Worked:** Back.
2. **Secondary Muscles Worked:** Middle back, shoulders, biceps.
3. **The Move:** Sitting on a cable row machine with your legs almost fully extended, bend at the waist and grasp the handle. With the handle in hand, sit straight up while pulling the handle toward your waist. It is important while you are pulling (rowing) the weight toward your waist to arch your back slightly and sit with your chest out and shoulders square.
4. **Tip:** Bring the bar or handles to your waist and keep your elbows close to your sides.

## One-Arm Rows

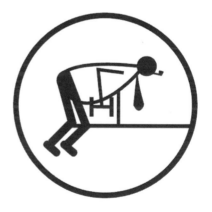

1. **Primary Muscles Worked:** Back.
2. **Secondary Muscles Worked:** Middle back, shoulders, biceps.
3. **The Move:** Rest one knee on a flat bench while keeping your other foot on the floor. With the arm that is on the side of the bench with your extended leg grasp a dumbbell parallel to your chest. Raise the dumbbell back toward your waist. Make sure to do this motion slowly and slightly arch your back.
4. **Tip:** The movement should feel like you are using an imaginary saw.

## Preacher Curls

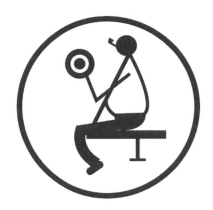

1. **Primary Muscles Worked:** Biceps.
2. **Secondary Muscles Worked:** Forearms.
3. **The Move:** Sitting on a preacher bench using a straight bar or curve bar, grasp the bar slightly wider than the elbows. Starting position should be with your arms 95 percent extended. From the starting position, curl with your biceps toward your chin. Hold for two seconds while flexing and return to the starting position.
4. **Tip:** Don't extend (lock out) your arms; this puts undo pressure on your tendons.

## Dumbbell Curls

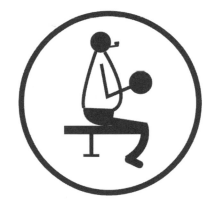

1. **Primary Muscles Worked:** Biceps.
2. **Secondary Muscles Worked:** Forearms.
3. **The Move:** Sitting or standing, grasp a dumbbell with each hand. Starting position, palms and weight should be at your sides. Slowly curl weight up while rotating palms upward toward your chest. Ending position, your palms should be facing you about eight inches parallel from your shoulders.
4. **Tip:** By rotating your palms from the starting position to the ending position, you isolate the biceps muscle.

## Concentration Curls

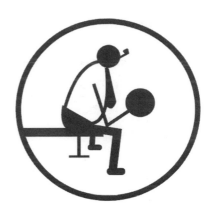

1. **Primary Muscles Worked:** Biceps.
2. **Secondary Muscles Worked:** Forearms.
3. **The Move:** Sitting on the edge of a bench, rest your elbow on the inside of your knee. Take a dumbbell and curl toward your face. Return to starting position near your ankle.
4. **Tip:** Palm should be facing up and motion should be slow and controlled.

## Cable Curls

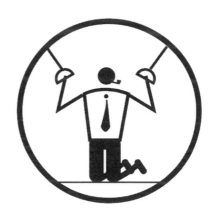

1. **Primary Muscles Worked:** Biceps.
2. **Secondary Muscles Worked:** Forearms.
3. **The Move:** Using a cable machine start with the pulley and handle in the upper position. Grasp handle and proceed to curl weight as if you were trying to flex like a bodybuilder.
4. **Tip:** Go slow and feel the biceps contract.

### Triceps Press Downs

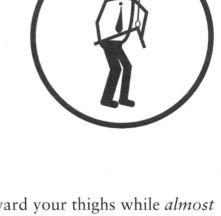

1. **Primary Muscles Worked:** Back of arm (Triceps).
2. **Secondary Muscles Worked:** Shoulders.
3. **The Move:** Stand at a cable machine with a V-shaped or curved handle that is positioned on the upper pulley. While standing upright, grasp the V-bar at chest level and press down toward your thighs while *almost* locking out your elbows. Use your elbows as a hinge and keep them close to your body. Do not lean into the weight for this is a triceps exercise, not an inverted shoulder press.
4. **Tip:** Keep your elbows tight to your body.

### Triceps French Press

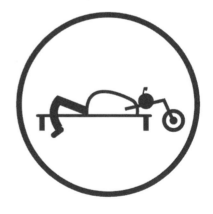

1. **Primary Muscles Worked:** Triceps.
2. **Secondary Muscles Worked:** Shoulders.
3. **The Move:** Laying on a bench grasp a barbell slightly closer than shoulder width apart. Hold the bar above you at chest level. Bend at your elbows letting your lower arms and the barbell lower toward your forehead. Raise back up to the starting position.
4. **Tip:** Go *slow* and use your elbows as a hinge.

## Triceps Kickbacks

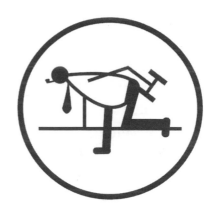

1. **Primary Muscles Worked:** Triceps.
2. **Secondary Muscles Worked:** None.
3. **The Move:** Start in the same position as one-arm rows. Take a light dumbbell and raise your elbow until it is parallel to the bench. Your forearm and fist should be pointing toward the floor. Gently (kick back) the dumbbell and forearm in the opposite direction of your upper body. Your elbow should not move, however you will feel tightness in the back of your arm. That is your triceps flexing during the movement. Return back to the starting position and repeat.
4. **Tip:** Use your elbow as a hinge, and do not swing your arm.

## Triceps Overhead Extensions

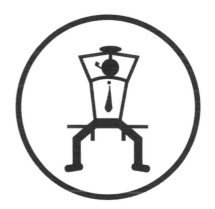

1. **Primary Muscles Worked:** Triceps.
2. **Secondary Muscles Worked:** Shoulders.
3. **The Move:** Sit upright on the edge of the bench with your feet flat on the floor. Grasp a dumbbell with either hand (or barbell) and raise the weight completely over your head and rest the weight behind your neck. Your elbows should be pointing toward the ceiling. Extend the weight while locking out your elbows above your head. Return to the starting position and repeat.
4. **Tip:** Point your elbows to the sky at all times.

### Leg Extensions

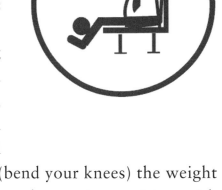

1. **Primary Muscles Worked:** Thighs (front).
2. **Secondary Muscles Worked:** Hips and hip abductors.
3. **The Move:** Start by sitting on a leg extension machine. Adjust pad at the ankle. Starting position, legs should be fully extended while your back remains pressed against the back rest. Lower (bend your knees) the weight about halfway down. Return to the starting position with knees locked out.
4. **Tip:** Going through a full range of motion will put undo stress on the knees, so please only lower the weight *halfway*.

### Leg Curls

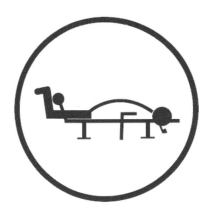

1. **Primary Muscles Worked:** Hamstrings (back of legs).
2. **Secondary Muscles Worked:** Calves.
3. **The Move:** Lie flat on your stomach on a leg curl machine. Place the curling pad at the back of your ankles. Slowly raise your heels toward your buttocks. Gently lower three-quarters of the way back to the starting position.
4. **Tip:** Keep waist firmly against the bench.

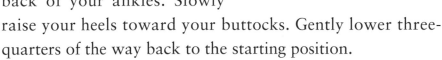

## Squats

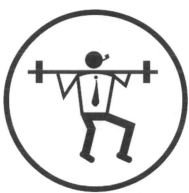

1. **Primary Muscles Worked:** Legs.
2. **Secondary Muscles Worked:** 50 percent of your body.
3. **The Move:** Standing straight with feet shoulder width apart, rest a barbell across the upper back. Start by lowering yourself into a squatting position by bending at the knees. Your thighs should never go below your knees, and return to the starting position.
4. **Tip:** When squatting down, fill your chest up with air, when pressing up exhale completely.

## Lunges

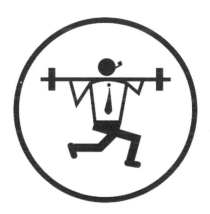

1. **Primary Muscles Worked:** Thighs, glutes (rear).
2. **Secondary Muscles Worked:** All of the legs.
3. **The Move:** Rest the weight on your shoulders. Start with legs shoulder width apart. Take a step forward (lunge) while keeping your knee perpendicular with your ankle. Gently touch your opposite knee to the floor and return to the starting position by pushing off your front foot.
4. **Tip:** Keep your back straight, abdominals tight, and concentrate on form.

Now that you understand the Fat Daddy weight workout, you probably have gathered that all of these new muscles will require a lot of energy (food) to maintain. That ties directly back to eating the right foods and the right amount of foods. For every pound of new muscle you add to your body, you will burn about sixty more calories per day. That can really add up; just look at the chart below:

| MUSCLE BURNS FAT | | |
| --- | --- | --- |
| **POUNDS OF NEW MUSCLE** | **POUNDS OF FAT BURNED PER MONTH** | **POUNDS OF FAT BURNED PER YEAR** |
| 1 | 0.5 | 6 |
| 3 | 1.5 | 19 |
| 5 | 2.6 | 31 |
| 10 | 5.1 | 62 |
| 12 | 6.2 | 74 |
| 15 | 7.7 | 93 |
| 20 | 10.3 | 123 |

By adding just ten pounds of muscle to your body, it will burn off sixty-two pounds of fat over one year. And it will keep burning those extra calories year after year. That means that when you've lost the fat, you can eat a lot more and not gain back the fat. (Although I still don't recommend chowing down a dozen doughnuts just yet.) Also, with less fat and more muscle, your body will have the lean, toned, fit look that every man aspires to.

Combining strength training, stretching, and cardio, you can transform your body without starving yourself on a low-calorie diet. And the most dramatic difference you'll probably see is right in the gut. So let's talk about some abdominal workouts.

## The Middle of Your Field—Your Abs

Does this sound familiar:

Loving Wife to Loving Husband: "Does my butt look big in this?"

Loving Husband to Loving Wife: "Yes, your butt looks big in everything. And my gut hangs over my button flys. But we're stuck together now, so who cares? Let's eat some pie."

Sound familiar? No, probably not. It's too honest. But, let's face it, as the women in our lives get older, they start worrying more and more about how wide their caboose looks. For dads like us, the problem is the beer gut and the love handles, also known as the Dunlop disease. Most try busting their guts by doing sit-ups and crunches. But if you're looking for washboard abs, 10 million crunches alone won't get you there. A defined midriff has more to do with the absence of belly fat and a diet very low in carbs and fat than it does with bulging stomach muscles. So don't expect to trim inches from your waistline by crunching them away.

Also, strong stomach muscles can help protect the spine during twisting and heavy lifting; many studies suggest that abdominal workouts only slightly reduce the risk of lower back pain. In fact, many researchers have found that several types of abdominal exercises—including leg lifts—put undue stress on the back and should be avoided.

The belly is actually broken up into four different muscle groups. There's the upper abs (rectus abdominus), lower abs, and the external and internal obliques. Sadly, there's no single exercise that's best for all of them.

To give your abs the best possible workout, you have to find several exercises that you can perform comfortably. Whatever workout you try for that growing gut, keep a slow, steady pace and stop at the first sign of pain. And those attorneys again insist on a warning: If you're recovering from a back injury or have pain, talk to your doctor about the exercises that are right for you. Now, here's a brief list of exercises that can help you strengthen your abdominals:

## Crunches (Upper and Middle Abs)

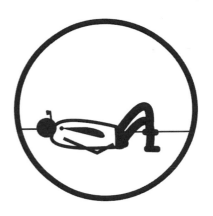

Lie down with your feet flat on the ground or resting on a bench or bed or couch or whatever. Cross your hands over your body or out to your sides. Roll your shoulders slightly toward your knees. Feel the contraction in your abdominals. Your back should remain pressed firmly against the ground at all times. The range of movement is only six to eight inches. Exhale completely when performing the crunching part of the exercise. Do fifteen or twenty reps, rest twenty seconds, and repeat.

## Toe Touches (Upper Abdominals)

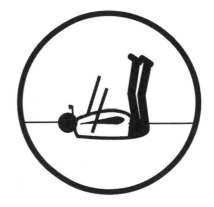

Lie on your back. With your legs and feet together, rise up at a 90-degree angle from your upper torso. Raise your arms straight above you toward your toes. Flex and squeeze your abdominals when rising toward your toes. Do fifteen or twenty reps, rest twenty seconds, and repeat.

## Cable Crunches (Upper Abs and Sides)

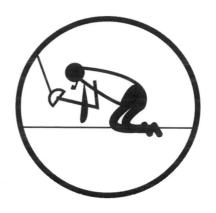

Get on your knees in front of a high-cable pulley with a rope attachment and grab both ends. Draw your hands down by the sides of your ears (palms facing in) or just above your forehead. Keeping your hands locked in place, slowly curl yourself down and forward, first drawing your chin toward your chest, then letting your shoulders and back follow. Curl yourself down as far as you comfortably can, then slowly reverse the motion back up. Do two sets of fifteen repetitions.

## Reverse Crunches (Lower Abs)

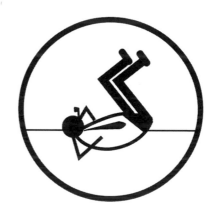

Lie faceup, knees bent, heels close to your butt, and fingertips behind your head. Without changing your knee angle, contract the abs to curl your tailbone a few inches off the floor, knees rolling toward your chest. Avoid moving your thighs to lift higher, and keep your heels toward buttocks. Slowly lower to the floor. Repeat the same movements for all reps. Begin with eight to twelve reps and gradually build to sixteen to twenty reps.

### Leg Raises (Lower Abs)

Sit on the end of a bench or on the ground. Anchor your hands firmly behind you. Straighten your legs in front of you while leaning back slightly. Slowly bend the knees toward your chest and lean forward. Your chest and knees should almost meet in the middle of your abdominal contraction. Hold the contraction for five seconds and release. Try to do twelve to fifteen repetitions.

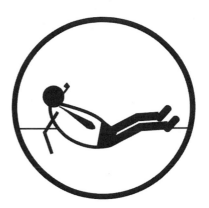

### The Plank (Sides and Overall Abs)

Extend your legs back and keep your feet together, so you're supported on your forearms and the balls of your feet. Hold for twenty seconds. Relax. Do three reps.

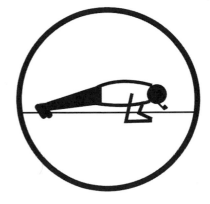

### Side Crunch (Obliques)

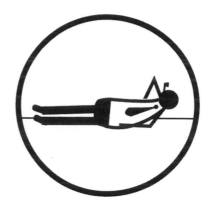

Lie on your side with your knees bent. Place one arm behind your head and the other arm out to your side for support. Slowly raise your upper body toward your knees. Focus on the muscle on the side of your torso. Flex and hold for three seconds. Release. Try to do twenty repetitions and two sets.

You need another couple tips for the best abdominal training. For one, make sure to contract and keep the tension on your abdominal muscles throughout the entire set. Even if you never land on the cover of *Playgirl*—and, seriously, let's hope you don't—you'll get a lot more out of your abdominal workouts this way. You'll also see that stronger stomach muscles can improve your posture while boosting your performance in a wide variety of sports. But remember, if you want to look better without your shirt, you will need to watch what, when, and how much you eat. And, also, you'll need to get your back waxed.

## Yoga

Many guys I know think yoga is for incense-burning, robe-wearing freaks who drink nothing but chai tea and love to chat about their proper place in the universe. And, yeah, there's some of that. But freaks are everywhere. You ever talk to a stripper? Did that keep you from going back to the nudie bar? No. So don't let a strange stereotype stop you from trying yoga. It is actually a great way to build strength, flexibility, and balance.

What's more, yoga, because it helps elongate muscles, is a good counterbalance to weight training workouts, which emphasize shortening muscles.

The word yoga means "to join or yoke together," and the practice dates back more than 5,000 years. I looked it up. It aims to bring the body and mind together in harmony. The whole system of yoga is built on three main structures: exercise, breathing, and meditation. Practicing yoga involves moving your body through a range of different types of isometric and stretching movements called "poses." The yoga poses emphasize extreme concentration. The focus is on holding the pose and controlling your breathing for sustained periods.

## The Popular Types of Yoga

■ **Hatha Yoga:** The "forceful yoga," or hatha yoga, was developed in medieval times. (I looked that up, too.) Hatha yoga uses different "poses," called asanas, to strengthen, open, and cleanse the body. These asanas can be categorized by the movement they create in the body. For example, there are forward bends (like touching the toes), back bends (looking up), twists (turning around), as well as inversions, standing, and sitting poses.

■ **Iyengar Yoga:** B. K. S. Iyengar was born in India on December 14, 1918. He studied hatha yoga as a youth and eventually developed his own particular style. He began teaching early on and soon became well known for his abilities. He's eighty-three today and is still a practicing yoga master. B. K. S. Iyengar's approach to yoga has been coined, coincidentally enough, "Iyengar yoga."

■ **Ashtanga Yoga:** This method involves a sequential order of correct breathing (Ujjayi Pranayama), poses (asanas), and gazing point (driste). "Ashtanga" literally means eight limbs. They are described by Patanjali as: Yama (abstinences), Niyama (observances), Asana (poses), Pranayama (breath control), Pratyahara (withdrawal of senses), Dharana (concentration), Dhyana (meditation), and Samadhi (contemplation). You don't need to remember all that, though. There won't be a quiz.

- **Bikram Yoga:** If you want to sweat, Bikram is for you. It's yoga done in a heated room to warm up your whole body. This allows you to work deep into your muscles, tendons, and ligaments and to change your body

> **ILLEGAL PROCEDURE**
>
> Yoga exercises are not recommended for children under sixteen because their bodies' nervous and glandular systems are still growing, and the effect of yoga exercises on these systems may interfere with natural growth. Children may safely practice meditation and simple breathing exercises as long as the breath is never held. These techniques can greatly help children learn to relax, concentrate, and reduce impulsiveness. Children trained in these techniques are better able to manage emotional upsets and cope with stressful events.

from the inside out. Bikram yoga is a process that can reduce the symptoms of many chronic diseases, and it is an excellent preventive activity for parts of the body that are healthy. There's a serious caution here. Many women practice this type of yoga in bikinis, while many men do this in Speedos. If there are going to be girls in bikinis around, you might want to skip the Speedos and bring some baggy shorts, if you get my, ah, point.

- **Power Yoga:** Power yoga combines many of the techniques from most yoga disciplines and is done very fast. It's a very hard workout.

### Upward-Facing Dog

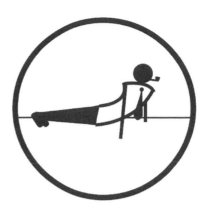

1. **Muscles Worked:** Lower back, abs, feet, chest.
2. **Starting Point:** Lying on your stomach.
3. **The Move:** Lie prone on the floor. Stretch your legs back, with the tops of your feet on the floor. Bend your elbows and spread your palms on the floor beside your waist so that your forearms are more or less perpendicular to the floor. Inhale and press your inner hands firmly into the floor and slightly back, as if you were trying to push yourself forward along the floor. Then straighten your arms and simultaneously lift your torso up and your legs a few inches off the floor on an inhalation. Keep the thighs firm and slightly turned inward, the arms firm and turned out so the elbow creases face forward. Press the tailbone toward the pubis and lift the pubis toward the navel. Narrow the hip points. Firm but don't harden the buttocks. Firm the shoulder blades against the back and puff the side ribs forward. Lift through the top of the sternum but avoid pushing the front ribs forward, which only hardens the lower back. Look straight ahead or tip the head back slightly, but take care not to compress the back of the neck and harden the throat.

### Downward-Facing Dog

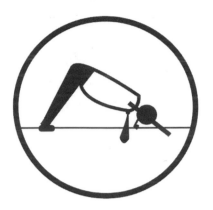

1. **Muscles Worked:** Shoulders, hamstrings, calves, arches, and hands.
2. **Starting Point:** Lying on your stomach.
3. **The Move:** Get down on your hands and knees. (Stop giggling.) Set your knees directly below your hips and your hands slightly forward of your shoulders. Spread your palms, index fingers parallel or slightly turned out, and turn your toes under. Exhale and lift your knees away from the floor. At first keep the knees slightly bent and the heels lifted away from the floor. Lengthen your tailbone away from the back of your pelvis and press it lightly toward the pubis. Against this resistance, lift the sitting bones toward the ceiling, and from your inner ankles draw the inner legs up into the groin. Then exhale and push your top thighs back and stretch your heels onto or down toward the floor. Straighten your knees but be sure not to lock them. Firm the outer thighs and roll the upper thighs inward slightly. Narrow the front of the pelvis.

## Chair Pose

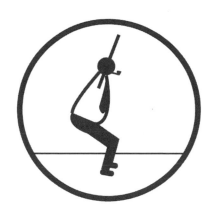

1. **Muscles Worked:** Thighs, lower back, shoulders, and arms.
2. **Starting Point:** Standing.
3. **The Move:** Standing straight up with your feet a little less than shoulder width apart and your arms at your sides—the yoga term for this is Tadasana. Inhale and raise your arms perpendicular to the floor. Either keep the arms parallel, palms facing inward, or join the palms. Exhale and bend your knees, trying to take the thighs as parallel to the floor as possible. The knees will project out over the feet, and the torso will lean slightly forward over the thighs until the front torso forms sort of a right angle with the tops of the thighs. Keep the inner thighs parallel to each other and press the heads of the thigh bones down toward the heels. Firm your shoulder blades against the back. Take your tailbone down toward the floor and in toward your pubis to keep the lower back long. Stay for thirty seconds to a minute. To come out of this pose straighten your knees with an inhalation, lifting strongly through the arms. Exhale and release your arms to your sides back into the standing position.

**Reverse Triangle Pose**

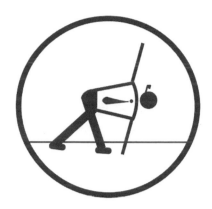

1. **Muscles Worked:** Legs, hips, chest, and back.
2. **Starting Point:** Standing.
3. **The Move:** Stand in Tadasana. Exhale, stepping or lightly jumping to put your feet three to four feet apart. Raise your arms parallel to the floor and reach them actively out to the sides, shoulder blades wide, palms down. Turn your left foot in 45 to 60 degrees to the right and your right foot out to the right 90 degrees. Align the right heel with the left heel. Firm your thighs and turn your right thigh outward, so that the center of the right kneecap is in line with the center of the right ankle. Exhale, turning your torso to the right, and square your hip points as much as possible with the front edge of your sticky mat. As you bring the left hip around to the right, resist the head of the left thighbone back and firmly ground the left heel. Exhale again, turning your torso further to the right and lean forward over the front leg. Reach your left hand down, either to the floor (inside or outside the foot) or, if the floor is too far away, onto a block positioned against your inner right foot. Allow the left hip to drop slightly toward the floor. You may feel the right hip slip out to the side and lift up toward the shoulder, and the torso hunch over the front leg. To counteract this, press the outer right thigh actively to the left and release the right hip away from the right shoulder. Use your right hand, if necessary, to create these two movements, hooking the thumb into the right hip crease. Beginners should keep their head in a neutral position, looking straight forward, or turn it to look at the floor.

More experienced practitioners can turn the head and gaze up at the top thumb. From the center of the back, between the shoulder blades, press the arms away from the torso. Bring most of your weight to bear on the back heel and the front hand. Stay in this pose anywhere from thirty seconds to one minute. Exhale, release the twist, and bring your torso back to upright with an inhalation. Repeat for the same length of time with the legs reversed, twisting to the left.

## Warrior II

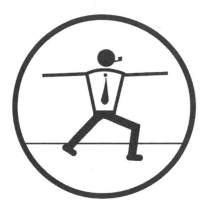

1. **Muscles Worked:** Legs, chest, shoulders, and arms.
2. **Starting Point:** Standing.
3. **The Move:** Stand in Tadasana. Exhale, stepping or lightly jumping to put your feet three and a half to four feet apart. Raise your arms parallel to the floor and reach them actively out to the sides, shoulder blades wide, palms down. Turn your right foot in slightly to the right and your left foot out to the right 90 degrees. Align the left heel with the right heel. Firm your thighs and turn your left thigh outward so that the center of the left kneecap is in line with the center of the left ankle. Exhale and bend your left knee over the left ankle, so that the shin is perpendicular to the floor. If possible, bring the left thigh parallel to the floor. Anchor this movement of the left knee by strengthening the right leg and pressing the outer right heel firmly to the floor. Stretch the arms away from the space between the shoulder blades, parallel to the floor. Don't lean the torso over the left

thigh: Keep the sides of the torso equally long and the shoulders directly over the pelvis. Press the tailbone slightly toward the pubis. Turn the head to the left and look out over the fingers. Stay for thirty seconds to one minute. Inhale to come up. Reverse the feet and repeat for the same length of time to the left.

## Changing Stadiums

Okay, you have concerns. I hear you. You're working, like, a lot, and you're not sure you can do an hour a day of exercise. It's understandable. The total time a man spends at work has increased 2.8 hours a week since 1977, according to the Families and Work Institute—from 47.1 hours to 49.9 hours. Those extra hours, and all those fatherly duties have you stretched thinner than Calista Flockhart. But your work and exercise don't have to be mutually exclusive. Working out is not only something you do in one or two defined periods each day. You can stick mini-workouts into your everyday routine. To wit:

- **Skip the elevator.** Aim to take the stairs at least three times every day. With just five minutes of stair climbing you'll burn 42 more calories than if you rode an escalator or elevator.

- **Take the long route.** If you leave your desk to go to the bathroom, take the stairs up to the bathroom on the next floor.

- **Stand at attention.** Each time your phone rings, stand up to take the phone call. Pace while you talk.

Now, let's be specific with some mini-exercises you can do at home, in traffic, on an airplane, in a meeting, wherever:

- **Chest Press:** Put your hands together under your chin as if you were "praying." Now squeeze your elbows together by tightening your chest. Hold for ten seconds and release.

- **Shoulder Raise:** Cross your hands in your lap by interlocking your fingers. Now try to raise your elbows up while your fingers stay tightly interlocked, and firmly resting in your lap.

- **Thigh Squeeze:** Straighten your legs in front of you as far as they will go. Tighten and squeeze the muscles in the front of your legs and hold for ten seconds.

- **Leg Extension–Curl Combo:** While sitting at your desk, place your left heel against your right toe. Slowly straighten out your right leg while pushing back against it and "resisting" the movement with your left leg. Once your leg is completely straight, reverse the movement: push back with your left leg and resist with your right leg until you have returned to the starting position. This exercise tones the muscles in the front of your thighs (quadriceps) as well as the muscles in the back of your thighs (hamstrings).

- **Squats:** Stand straight up from your chair, taking care not to lock your knee into a full straightened position or overarch your lower back. As you do so, squeeze or "contract" your buttocks. At the top of the motion, squeeze the buttocks even tighter and slowly sit back down, touching your buttocks only lightly to the chair before you stand back up into the next repetition. Hint: Do this as many times per day as you stand up! When you stand to take a phone call, incorporate a squat at the beginning, middle, and end of the call. This move helps tone the buttocks and legs.

- **Rows:** Sitting up as tall as possible, with your feet on the floor, grab the edge of your desk with an underhand grip and with both hands. If your chair has wheels, make sure that it's far enough away from your desk that your arms are just slightly bent. Pull yourself in toward your desk until your elbows are just slightly behind your waist. Press outward and straighten your arms out to the start. (If your chair does not have wheels, start with your arms bent at a little more than 90 degrees. Plant your feet into the floor, and just pull on the desk for a slow count of three as if you were trying to move it towards you. Relax between repetitions.) This move tones your upper back and arms.

- **Wall Push-Ups:** Stand about an arm's length away from a wall, with your palms pressed against it and your feet about hip width apart. Bend your elbows and let your body move toward the wall. Once your elbows are bent to about 90 degrees, straighten your arms and return to the start. This move strengthens your chest, shoulders, and arms.

- **Seated Crunches:** Sit up tall with one hand behind your head and the other one holding onto the edge of your chair's seat. Pull your abdominal muscles inward. Slowly curl down and forward just a few inches. As you do so, pull your abs in even tighter. Hold a moment and then slowly uncurl to a very tall position. This move strengthens your abdominal muscles.

- **Chair Dips:** While sitting at your desk, try doing "chair dips." This is for the triceps on the back of your upper arm. Begin by placing your palms on your armrests, and push yourself up out of your chair. (Be careful if your chair has wheels or is unsteady.) Initially, you should use your legs to help offset the resistance. As you get stronger, you can rely less on your legs and more on your arms. Perform fifteen repetitions. Do only one set to start, then gradually work up to two or three sets of fifteen repetitions as you become more fit.

■ **Desk Push-Ups:** From a standing position, you could do a modified "desk push-up." This will work your triceps, along with your chest and shoulders. Put your arms on the edge of the desk and then walk your feet back until your body is straight. Lower yourself toward the desk so that your chest nearly touches it. Push back up until your arms are straight. (This activates considerably more muscle fibers than the chair dips, so don't do too many to start or you'll be sore for days!) Try one set of fifteen repetitions and see how you feel the next day.

■ **Arm Curls:** For your biceps muscles, any type of arm-curl exercise will be beneficial. For example, you might use something like a briefcase, or anything else with a handle. Perform the curl with your elbow close to your side. This will help reduce the overall strain on your lower back and maximize the workout on your biceps muscles. For a good isometric (static-type) exercise, when seated in front of your desk, reach your arms forward and grasp the under portion of the top of your desk with both hands (palms up); then, slowly and steadily, pull against that resistance and hold for about six seconds. Repeat four or five times.

■ **Chair Squats:** For the legs and hips, you might want to try a basic squat movement. You could actually do what are called "chair squats." It's as simple as going from the seated to standing position and repeating this movement for fifteen repetitions. Keep your feet about shoulder width apart, and lower yourself to no less than 90 degrees at the knee. You may have to adjust your seat height accordingly.

■ **Calf Raises:** While standing in the copier room waiting for 200 double-sided sheets to print, try some calf raises. All you have to do is lift yourself up onto your toes. Repeat fifteen times.

Take a breather and repeat. You may be able to tolerate more sets on this one since you use your calves with every step you take. But still, be careful not to overdo it, or you'll know about it for a few days!

Additionally, like every good athlete, you should stretch throughout the day, not just at the gym. In fact it's pretty easy to stretch at your desk. Fat Daddy recommends that you stretch every three hours or so for just a few minutes to get the kinks out. Some basic stretches to do at your desk:

■ Separate your knees and slowly lean forward. Try to keep your back flat as you try to touch your chest to your thighs. Breathe normally and hold twenty seconds.

■ Stretch your shoulders and neck by gently rolling your shoulders clockwise and counter clockwise ten times in each direction.

■ Stretch your lower back by draping forward over your lap.

■ To stretch the back of your leg, extend your leg, lean over in your chair and reach your arms towards your feet. You can increase the effectiveness of this stretch by lifting your toe up in the air. (Repeat on both sides.)

## Extra Point

If you "just do it" you'll do "it" more. In 1990 there was a study done by the University of San Diego that followed seventy-eight inactive sedentary men. During a nine-month study, these sedentary men were given moderate exercise plans to follow—everything from walking to stair climbing. The men kept journals of their sexual activity before and after the study. After nine months on the program the *average* increase in sexual activity was around 30 percent, ranging from passionate kissing to intercourse or masturbation.

Here's another study. Phillip Whitten, Ph.D., a behavioral scientist at Bentley College in Waltham, Massachusetts, evaluated the sexual activity of 160 swimmers between the ages of forty and eighty. The majority of these aquatic exercisers had sex lives more active than people twenty years their junior.

So you're asking, "What's the relationship between exercise and sex?" Well, researchers note a spike in brain wave activity. It changes drastically after you start working out. They figure this means men who exercise feel more energized and focused. Also, their body temperatures rise, which is also one of the main sensations associated with arousal. Still, you don't want to "just do it" too much. Excess physical activity can cause the libido to wither. If you run fifty miles a week or have a strenuous workout every day you're probably hurting your sex drive instead of helping it.

A couple final points here about exercise. Taking the first step is the hardest. But once you start, stick with it. After a few weeks, what once seemed hard will seem easy. When that happens, call time-out and reevaluate your game plan. Focus on frequency, duration, and intensity. Then get back in the game and step up the exercise program. You'll see even more progress.

Also, exercise in the morning. You'll burn more calories, and you'll probably stick with your exercise program longer. If you decide to exercise at lunch or late in the afternoon, you're giving yourself more time to invent excuses about why you can't exercise. Don't give yourself the chance to dog it.

## PLAYBOOK NOTES: Fitness—The Framework

1. Quitters never win, and winners never quit. If you start, you have to stick with it.

2. Know the proper etiquette and lingo before you hit the gym.

3. Stretch—a lot!

4. Follow a four quarters workout. Stretching, weights, cardio, yoga.

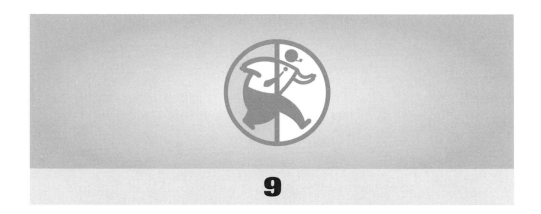

# 9

# Family—The Fundamentals

"Coaches should build men first and football players second."
— EDDIE ROBINSON, former Head
Coach of Grambling University

### Being a Father, and Father Time

It was Monday morning. I'd had a weekend full of kid-friendly activities, culminating with my daughter being up all Sunday night with an ear infection and with me getting three hours of sleep. I had slept through the alarm as a result. At 6 A.M. I was already running late.

Still, I went to the gym. Spent an hour trying to wake up between sets, rode the bike, stretched, and then stumbled to the showers. Two nicks and cuts later, it was off to work. At my desk by 8:00, meetings until 2:00, client visit at 3:00, conference call at 5:00, executive staff meeting at 5:30, administrative cleanup at 6:00, in the car headed home for dinner at 6:30.

And that's when it hit me: I've been lied to. Fooled. Tricked. Hornswoggled. Remember on *Bewitched* when Derwood, er, Darin came home? His wife greeted him with a kiss and a martini. A freaking martini! Then that little witch daughter of theirs, Tabitha, came running up and gave Darin a kiss. And somehow Darin never spilled a drop of his drink. When Fred MacMurray came home in *My Three Sons*, he said his hellos, donned a sweater, and plopped down in a cozy chair to read the evening paper. Fatherhood was nice and easy and contained a nice whiff of juniper berries. Right? TV couldn't be wrong? It had to be like that.

Except it isn't. There's no evening paper, no martinis. Just, "Dad, play with me." "Look what I made you at school." "Can I have a dog?" "Teacher says I have lice."

And that's before you even get through the doorway. On a good day you can make it to the dinner table a half hour later. But then it's all, "Stop playing with your food." "Leave your sister alone." "Leave your brother alone." "Don't play with your food." After dinner it's time for homework and matching cows with moos and farmers with tractors. Then comes baths and the "time for bed" agreement—something that is as fuzzy and binding as the Geneva Convention.

Eventually it is 9:30, the kids are asleep, you're beat, and where the hell is my martini?

Maybe I knew it wouldn't really be like TV. Maybe not. But I'm not sure any of us realizes what we're really in for. Both ends of fatherhood—the constant demands, the incredible responsibilities, and, yes, the real joy of having kids—are really hard to explain.

That's why I wanted to make sure Fat Daddy spoke to dads from a dad. Most of the books that were available to me as both a new (and now seasoned) father just helped me to be a more supportive husband. If I wanted to be a titan of industry, I had plenty of books to choose from. If I wanted to be a better lover, there were four aisles of books and that one dingy video store on the other side of town where I could seek knowledge. To manage my workout and diet there was also no shortage of information—from Atkins to the Zone to the fitness segments on that Kelly and Regis show (she's so cute and he's so wacky!) and everything in between. But how could I do it all? How could I be a real dad, eat right, work out, and treat my spouse well? A book on that certainly wasn't readily available.

I looked everywhere and found nothing. Nada. Zip.

So I wrote it myself. And, despite all the words that have come so far and the ones you've still yet to read, there is a way to simplify this whole book. There are two principles. One: time management. Two: priorities.

Maybe that's too simple. Maybe not. But in this mommy-dominated world, I felt "manly men" were ready for a Fat Daddy type of book. That's why Fat Daddy is for all types of dads: black, white, Asian, and Hispanic dads. Single dads, widowed or divorced dads, Jewish dads, and Christian dads. Homosexual dads to heterosexual dads. Bottom line, us dads share a common bond—we need to find balance in that period after we stop being boys and become dads. We need to manage our time well and match that with our priorities (see . . . well, you get the idea) for taking care of not just our families but our own bodies and minds. That's the goal. And you don't have to reach it alone. That's where Fat Daddy comes in.

## Good Dad, Bad Dad

You, my friend, are probably getting rounder, less appealing to your mate, and unhealthier on the inside. Not that there's anything wrong with that. Maybe you like that bowling ball under your shirt. Maybe you like having your own boobs.

Or maybe you're not quite that bad yet. Maybe you're a more subtle kind of unhealthy. Take the case of a friend of mine. He had a cardiac arrest at his desk not that long ago. Bang. He didn't even spill his coffee. (Sudden cardiac arrest, by the way, kills over 250,000 Americans each year). At his memorial service I listened to people eulogize how much he helped others, how gracious he was, and what a good father he was. Then, in a weird and almost spiritual way, I found myself pondering the "father" comment. I'd known the man for a number of years, and I knew he certainly wasn't a bad father—but a good father? Was this real praise, or simply an acknowledgment that he'd had three kids? He smoked like a burning oil well, drank like a sailor on leave, and kicked it before he was fifty. Was that what a good father would do?

"It's an interesting question," says Dr. Jeffrey Whitman, a father of three girls in Dallas. "Not so long ago being a good dad meant being a good provider, a firm disciplinarian (when spankings didn't result in Child Protective Services making a visit at your front door), and staying out of mom's way. But now, being a good father means so much more—like helping mom actually raise the kids, doing car pool, cleaning the house, and setting a good healthy example for your kids."

So I guess you could say that prepping for fatherhood is more than reading Dr. Spock, childproofing the electrical outlets, and buying a tiny baseball glove. That's the easy stuff. The harder stuff is doing what you need to do to live a healthy, long life where you're around for your kids as long as possible and where your kids learn to live healthy, long lives, too. See, if dads practice good healthy habits, kids will be more likely to have healthy habits too. And while that seems simple and obvious, only 24 percent of adults regularly exercise, and 65 percent are overweight. What gives?

# Fat Daddy Syndrome

Guys really never grow up, and we know it. We are reminded daily that we are still boys, still pigs, and still running our offense under the *Original Game Plan*. The older we get, though, the better we get at disguising our hedonistic ways. You still eat that cold, three-day-old pizza for breakfast. But now you store it in a plastic baggie in the refrigerator instead of just leaving the box on the floor of your apartment. But while you can hide some things, fat can't be concealed. More food, more stress, more responsibility, and no time for fitness or the family will make for an all-out blitz of blubber hanging over our belts. And it isn't just a physical problem. It is emotional as well. Me, I never saw it coming. Either time.

First, there was the bathing suit incident at the mall. It was a shocker, but I dealt with it, got rid of the fat, and climbed back on the fitness wagon pretty easily. Unfortunately, I fell right back off again when Mrs. Right and I had our second child. Back again with the love handles, growth in my gut, and two more belt notches in the

---

"How has my life changed? Well, 190 lbs. to 252 lbs., no basketball except for watching the occasional Lakers game or March Madness. More stress, making more money, spending more money, less time (for anything), less head hair, more nose, ear, and ass hair. More stress (did I already say more stress?). Less spontaneous sex time, more two-cookie sex (give the kids two cookies and lock the door). I go to bed at 8:30 p.m. wake up at 10:00 p.m., go to sleep at 11:00 p.m. to 2:00 a.m., and wake up religiously at 6:00 to 6:45 a.m., or whatever time my three-year-old gets me up. More stress, I think I mentioned that. Less beer, more vodka. 34-inch waist to a 38/40/42 depending upon the designer. Knee surgery because I was trying to walk with too much weight. I have regressed to cartoons, Sponge Bob, and Rug Rats. I think the old me is buried somewhere in my kids toy box."

—DAN HINKLE, a dad from San Clemente, California

wrong direction. How is a guy supposed to endure doughnut holes every day and not get fat?

Fat Daddy Syndrome is not rare. As a matter of fact, it is more the rule than the exception (it looks a lot like the "sneak" we discussed back in the second quarter, but this time you know it's coming). Problem is, many dads tend to throw in the towel when they start to grow because they just can't establish the discipline again when No. 2 arrives. The added stress can make most fathers become overwhelmed and resort to more food, more work, and more excuses. If this happens, it's game over. Unfortunately, this behavior for us parents is *the* most serious threat to the health of our children. If we don't set a good example we can bet our kids will grow up fat, unhealthy, and pass their bad habits down to generations to come.

## No Prizes for Second Place—Dads and Disease

Have you ever thought about the traditions and practices that you've inherited from your family? It's a cathartic exercise to make a list of the healthy habits that you picked up from your childhood. Okay, so maybe health and fitness were not as widely understood thirty years ago as they are today. But back then there were also not as many fried chicken nuggets or super-sized meals floating around.

And kids in those days ran around the neighborhood from dusk to dawn to get their exercise. Today, kids are in school longer, watching more TV, and sitting at the computer endlessly. And more than that is doing our kids and ourselves in. With the exception of a spike during the oil shock in the 1970s, food prices have dropped by an average of 0.2 percent per year—when adjusted for inflation—since World War II, according to the Bureau of Labor Statistics. At the same time, the average American food intake, which was 1,826 calories per day in the 1970s is now around 2,100 calories per day. That's more than a 10 percent increase. Couple this with those massive fast-food portions (original McDonald's fries have about 200 calories, while a super-size order has about 600), and we not only have Fat Daddies, but fat families.

| HAPPY MEAL? | |
| --- | --- |
| **SCHOOL LUNCH** | **FAST FOOD** |
| Roasted chicken, corn on the cob, roll, orange, chocolate milk | Cheese burger, small french fry, small cola |
| 635 calories | 690 calories |
| 17% calories from fat | 32% calories from fat |
| 7.2% saturated fat | 21% saturated fat |
| *Source: City of New York Office of School Food and Nutrition Services* | |

This brings me back to my friend who is pushing up tulips. His family is suffering for his neglect of proper nutrition and exercise. And the suffering may not stop soon. He didn't set a good example for his kids in this area, so the only way they will learn the value of proper diet and exercise is from mom, or on their own—if at all. So, was he a good father? Well, okay, I really think he was. But his unexpected death was also partly his fault. The moral of the story is simple. Our mortality is directly correlated to how healthy we are. Heart disease, diabetes, colorectal and prostate cancer, and even depression are connected to what's on our plate and how often we exercise. We can help ourselves live longer and in the process we can help our kids and their kids live longer and healthier, too.

So put these tips in your playbook for a better life.

## Health and Wellness Sure Play—The Lucky 7

1. **Get tested.** If caught early, most cancer fatalities can be mitigated when caught in a treatable stage.

2. **Eat your colors.** Green, yellow, and red vegetables as well as many fruits are loaded with photochemicals and fiber that help fight free radicals and disease. (This daddy likes broccoli, blueberries, tomatoes, and yellow peppers.)

3. **Drink only in moderation.** One to two glasses of red wine or spirits per day. That's it. No beer bongs. No shots. Grow up.

4. **If you smoke or dip—quit.**

5. **Move it.** If you work out, great. If you don't, start. The Institute for American Cancer Research recommends one hour per day. If you can't do the full hour, at least take the stairs at work.

6. **Wear sunscreen.** There are over 1 million cases of skin cancer reported every year. If you go outside for any reason, wear a minimum of SPF 15. I like Cetaphil; it's a daily moisturizer and sunscreen in one. Doesn't stink, isn't slimy, and has SPF 30.

7. **Scrape the char.** You're a dad, so you're the master of the grill. So you should know that when protein (steaks, chicken, or fish) are exposed to high heat for too long they char. That char has many carcinogens. The crusty stuff may be tasty, but scrape it off if you want to live to grill another day.

## Team Captains

Having children changes your life, no doubt about it. But first, it changes your days, your hours, and your minutes. From the moment you know your Mrs. Right is pregnant, the two-minute drill begins. You count months before delivery, then minutes between contractions. Then suddenly you're counting the hours between feedings and naps. Soon you'll be counting time-outs, school days, and curfews. And sometimes, you'll be saying, "I'm going to count to three. . . ."

Just knowing where your time goes isn't enough. You also need to separate the activities you're enjoying from those you're not. Then, decide which of the unenjoyable tasks are really necessary (e.g., family, exercise, and job). Researchers at the Strong Families Study—an ongoing, international survey of 14,000 families that's been conducted over twenty years—found that many parents regularly overcommitted themselves to things they didn't like to do. The strongest families recognized this sad fact only after they made a list of the tasks that made their lives seem hectic. "Inevitably they found activities that weren't important, that they didn't have to do, and that didn't make them happy," says Nick Stinnett, Ph.D., lead researcher in the study and a professor of human development and family studies at the University of Alabama. "So they simply stopped doing them." Being more selective (such as not going to every PTA meeting) creates free hours and relieves a great deal of stress.

Most dads are already pros at doing two or even three things at once. This isn't a bad idea, as long as you realize that some combinations are better than others. You can combine daily exercise with spending time with a friend, if both of you like to walk or play squash. But taking a toddler out to dinner while trying to get conversation time in with your spouse is probably a bad idea. Your toddler's goal—to have your attention—directly conflicts with your desire to talk to your partner. Also, kids have no idea what to do with an oyster fork.

Still, you can combine spending time with your children, with, say, spring cleaning. In fact, the time spent on this kind of combined task may actually be better than things that are planned exclusively around children. Family chores also give parents an opportunity to communicate with their team. Just remember, finding time for family shouldn't be an afterthought or an item on your to-do list. As a team captain, eating better and exercising will not only do wonders for your family health, but will bring you closer together.

Sum it all up with these two certainties:

**Given 2.1:** Having a baby changes your life. Duh.

**Given 2.2:** To have a successful marriage you have to work as a team (or together as team *captains).*

## What's a Fat Family to Do?

"D-A-A-A-A-A-AAAAD," my son says, stretching the vowel until it breaks. "I'm bo-ored, I want to do something."
If I said, "let's go work out" he would have a meltdown.

In this case, it is time to lie. Okay, no, don't lie. Lying is bad, especially if you get caught. Let's say you shouldn't lie about fitness but you shouldn't be afraid to "sneak" it into your family life. When buying toys for your kids, select ones that require active participation—tyke bikes, push toys, climbing structures for toddlers; sports equipment, roller skates, jump ropes for older children. Leisure-time events can also be planned around active recreation—a backpacking trip, a day hike at a local park, or perhaps a bicycle or walking tour of your neighborhood. Your family will have so much fun; they probably won't even realize that they're getting fit. Just come up with a list of different fitness activities that your family could enjoy together and get to it.

Remember, though, there are some definite do's and don'ts when you are starting to get your family back into the fitness swing.

## The Do's

■ **Make it fun.** As with anything else in life, variety is the key to making your Fat Daddy family fitness program enjoyable. Exercising to the same Tae Bo tape every day isn't likely to hold an eight-year-old's attention, but weekly trips to the local swimming pool, rollerblading arena, and indoor baseball diamond likely will. You look for variety in your workout routine, so you take equal care to ensure there is variety in your family's plan.

■ **Start by encouraging your children when they are young to make physical activity a regular part of their day.** While playing organized sports is always a good way to stay fit as a family, don't limit yourselves to just football, baseball, basketball, and other ball games. Tossing a Frisbee around on a Sunday afternoon is a great way to get started. Maybe the whole family can take karate lessons at the local YMCA. Or combine household chores and exercise. Hold contests to see who can sweep the carpets the fastest, or wax the floors, or rake the leaves. You walk the dog every evening, why not walk the family? A simple daily walk around the neighborhood is one of the most relaxing, yet helpful, exercises in which a family can participate. Give everyone responsibility around the house, such as cleaning floors or raking leaves. Anything that gets the heart pumping faster is beneficial. Find something, *anything*, that holds everyone's interest and will make it easier to sustain an active lifestyle.

■ **Be supportive of your children and teens, regardless of their fitness level.** Just because your football coach thought the best way to motivate you was through insults doesn't mean it's the best way for you to coach your home team. And even if your teenager responds to every request from you with "Whatever," that doesn't mean you can be equally dismissive. Again, being a Fat

Daddy means not taking the easy, lazy way out. Shaming an overweight family member, especially children, is counterproductive and could be psychologically damaging. Listen to your kids' preferences and wishes and be sensitive to their degree of comfort and their ability level. Whether they participate in individual or group sports or totally do their own thing, be sure to encourage their interests and unique personality.

- **Eat dinner as a family.** Make a pleasant sit-down dinner a priority, at least a few nights a week. Encourage open, caring communication. Save the lectures for later; otherwise, children try to leave the table sooner and associate eating with high stress. Dinner should not be a chore.

- **Be a supportive role model.** For fitness to become a family value, we as parents have to set the example. You don't have to be Mr. Fitness to do so, but neither should you be attached to the couch with the remote five hours a night. If every request for fitness to your family is followed by a bratwurst belch, you will be tuned down. Make an effort to show the way. Lead. Support.

- **Make sure the activities are ones that everyone can participate in.** Choose things that fit your family's lifestyle and interests. No motorcross training for the third-grader, please.

- **Be flexible with scheduling.** Don't make it a "do or die" activity, and take into account that sometimes schedules change at the last minute. Enlist the kids to help you decide the best, most fun way to make up the exercise time lost. Look at interruptions as an *opportunity* to change up the routine, not a hindrance.

- **Encourage each other.** When someone in your family does something new, for example swimming a lap around the pool without stopping, give them a high five and a hearty "well done!"

When kids feel good about what they are doing, they'll keep it up and set new goals for themselves.

- **Keep a log of your family's fitness activities.** You'll find that if you do, everyone will want to join in and track their individual progress as well as find new ways for the family to stay fit together. This is the easiest part of the plan to ignore, but it is one of the most important. If you don't chart your progress, it's too easy to let the program deteriorate into vapor. You need a box score to check out how you're doing and where you're going.

- **You don't have to spend a lot of money to become physically fit and healthy as a family.** It just takes willpower, the motivation to say "yes" instead of "later." Wealthy people aren't fit because they pay money to a gym. *Anyone* who is fit is so because he or she has made a commitment, whether it be to a $200-a-month gym or to jogging through the neighborhood.

Bottom line, as the reformed Fat Daddy of the house, you need to always make exercise fun and enjoyable for everyone. And just like parenting, you have to be *consistent*.

## The Don'ts

- **Don't eat junk.** Parents often lecture their children about eating healthy but fill the kitchen cupboards with high-fat, sugary, salty, processed foods that offer no real nutritional value. Yeah, after work, there's nothing better than a cold beer and nine handfuls of mixed nuts. But again, you're not just cheating yourself when you do this, you're cheating your family, too. And it's not just the junk food you have in the house. Even the nutritional content of local school cafeteria food is highly questionable.

Driving through the Golden Arches is certainly easier than making a healthy, balanced dinner. But at what price? Certainly, an occasional treat or holiday overindulgence is fine, but as a daily habit, this kind of diet decreases immunity and reduces academic performance. The fact that life is hectic *is not an excuse*. Plan ahead. Make tough, disciplined decisions. It takes a committed effort to feed your family a healthy, balanced diet.

■ **Don't make the TV a baby-sitter.** Children and teens are bombarded by messages from peers and television that contribute to a sedentary "couch potato" mentality and lifestyle. Just take a look at the steady stream of television propaganda—steaming-hot pepperoni pizzas bubble over with melted cheese, your favorite sports superstar promises fun times from drinking a fizzy soda, rail-thin supermodels sashay across the television screen hawking, well, everything. Is it any wonder that our young people are confused about health and fitness? In moderation, TV and video games can be a fun form of easy entertainment—and, okay, Cartoon Network and the Disney Channel can be as addicting to Fat Daddies as it is to their munchkins—but in excess, it can give your child the wrong messages about good nutrition.

■ **Don't use food to punish or reward your child.** Withholding food can create fear in a child, leading to overeating later. If sweets are used as a reward, then children assume these foods are more valuable than other foods. And if you equate food with love, that could be setting your child up for food addiction.

■ **Don't be competitive.** With family fitness, there is no winner or loser. It should be fun, plain and simple. This is not your buddy on the golf course, this is your family. Don't make bets on weight loss or muscle gain.

Just remember, working out with the entire family isn't always the easiest thing to do, but once you start to make it part of your family's weekly routine, it will be part of who your family is—and that's the goal.

## The Plays

I'm not going to sugarcoat it. Exercise can be boring. So you have to keep changing it up, especially when you involve the whole family. If walking is one of your regular activities, turn the walk into an adventure for the kids. Have them pick a theme for the walk, like "space pirates" or "kid detectives." Then act out your theme while you walk. But, no costumes, please. This isn't a parade. You can also try to make fitness a subtle, rather than overt, part of your family's lifestyle.

### Preseason (The Easy Stuff)

- **Walk around the neighborhood.** Family walks are good bonding times. You can talk about important stuff while you stroll around. Be attuned to possible "teachable moments." When the children are young, push them in the stroller or pull a wagon in case they get tired of walking. Empower your kids by having a different child choose the route each time. It's also fun to choose an activity for each walk, such as pointing out different wildlife creatures or going on a doggy hunt (whoever spots the most dogs gets to read an extra bedtime story). Even as children get older, encourage them to walk with you. You may find a whole new world just around the corner.

- **Head for the park.** Remember in the movie *Arthur* when Arthur told Bitterman, "Take us through the park. You know how I love the park." Well, he was a big kid. A big, drunk kid, sure.

But still a kid, and kids love playing in the park. It's fun, and it is also a way to stay healthy through swinging, sliding, climbing, and so forth.

- **Rake leaves.** Raking leaves burns 300 calories in an hour! And when you're done, you can jump in them! That probably burns calories, too. But who cares?

- **Go for a walk indoors.** Don't skip your walk just because the weather's bad outside. Take your family fitness program indoors! You can either walk around your local mall or head for some spot that's a little more inspiring: even strolling through a museum can be a fitness activity. It doesn't matter what you're doing while you're walking, as long as you're moving quickly enough to get some benefits out of your workout.

- **Walk to school.** If you live close enough to your child's school, try walking instead of driving. You could form a daily or weekly walking group consisting of your child's neighborhood friends and his or her parents.

- **Anything outside.** Get out. Seriously. One activity out of the house, away from the office, and somewhere outside of the minivan with your family will inspire you to do more.

## Regular Season (Moderate)

If by now you feel that you won't be out of breath after the mad dash to the fridge at a commercial break, here are a few more fun family fitness ideas:

- **Play tag.** For variety, play "Flashlight Tag." All you need is a flashlight and a safe, dark area. We use our front yard. The object of the game is to avoid being hit by the light. Whoever is "it" shines the flashlight around until the light shines on another player. The one who gets caught in the light is "it." It's like laser tag, except without the lasers or all the dorks in the Battlestar Gallactica gear.

- **Use the wheels.** Bikes and rollerblades are fun ways to build family fitness. When our kids were younger, we pushed the stroller while skating. It is a great upper body workout. Now we all skate together. Bike riding on trails, in parks, and in your neighborhood is also a good option. In-line skate parks may make you feel old, though, unless you like wearing your britches around your thighs. Instead, find an old-school roller rink with a disco ball just like you went to in junior high. Okay, so that'll make you feel old, too. But at least your pants won't fall off.

- **Play ball.** Not dodge ball, of course. Yes, you'll beat your kids at it, but you'll also have to pay the dental bills when their teeth get knocked out. That's just no fair. Try kickball or a regular game of catch.

- **Hit the pool.** Few exercises will give you and your family as good a workout as swimming. Kids love it because they're not sweating, so they don't even think it's exercise.

- **Horseback riding.** Find a local stable that offers family rides. It's a workout for the horse, sure, but also for you. Riding a horse builds leg and arm strength and works on overall balance. Plus, your business will buy the old mare a little extra time before it heads off to the glue factory.

## The Playoffs (Fun and Fit!)

Okay, now for the really good stuff! If your family is now on the fitness wagon, try these activities. And remember, this is your family, not the Dallas Cowboys. You can lose without getting mad about it.

- **Running.** Sign up for a fun run or a 10k. It will be good for you and will benefit a good cause (also, you can use the cause as a way to teach your kids about social responsibility). But be sensitive to everyone in the family—don't sprint away from them just because you can. Check as well to see that everyone has proper running shoes.

- **Plan an adventure vacation.** Think "active" when planning a family vacation with older children and preteens. Call your travel agent for suggested adventure locations or plan your own trip. Include hiking, canoeing, rock climbing, white-water rafting, camping, horseback riding, biking, or skiing as a part of your vacation. Ask each family member to plan a day. You probably don't have to go far from home to experience the excitement of outdoor play as a family.

- **Skiing.** Seasons (and family funds) permitting, try cross-country skiing. Bring some hot chocolate and other snacks to make it a fun outing.

- **Canoeing.** Be sure to follow all safety rules, and make sure everyone wears a life preserver. This isn't your college white-water rafting trip. No coolers full of adult beverages, please.

- **Dancing.** Have your children teach you the latest dance craze. It will not only be a great workout for you, but your kids will get a great abdominal workout as their tummy clenches with riotous laughter. And you show you're a good sport. (Just don't let your buddies see.) Or you could always enroll in a class at your local Y or community center. What Fat Daddy's wife wouldn't want their man to get thinner while getting better on the dance floor?

- **Aerobics.** Rent an aerobic exercise tape from your local video store, or enroll in a class. Just don't fall into the trap of making this your only exercise, or you'll get bored fast. And if you take a class, don't choose it based on the hotness of the instructor. You're not there to exercise that muscle.

- **Ice-skating.** Using an established indoor or outdoor rink is the safest way to go. Check to see if they offer any discounts for families or groups. You'll be surprised how much you sweat on ice.

- **Rollerblading.** Remember to have everyone wear helmets, knee pads, and elbow pads to avoid injuries. Check local ordinances if you're going somewhere that's not a designated skate park.

## Babies and Fitness

It isn't easy to find an activity that appeals to kids, adults, and babies alike, but it is possible. Parents of young infants can buy a front pack to carry the baby. As the baby ages and can hold his head up, switch to a backpack kiddy chair. These kiddy harness packs allow you to walk briskly, hike, and even hold the leash of the family pooch. Always wear them with good posture. You may also want to invest in a jogging stroller, which can also be used for walking. They even navigate well on sand, dirt, and trails. There are also sturdy and stable strollers that attach to the back of your bike if you want to take your infant cycling with you; it's a great way for both of you to see the scenery.

Here's a sampling of ways to work out with your babies:

- **Kangaroo Walk:** Put your child in a baby carrier/jogger and take a walk. You can skip or hop when you're pushing the jogger. But try not to do so if people are watching. For a tougher workout, run behind a jogging stroller or hike some challenging hills.

- **Workout Video:** Pick up a mom-and-infant video.

- **Track Time:** Take your baby to a school track. If they are very young, spread out a blanket and bring some toys for them to play with while you walk or jog around them. Bring sand toys if there's a sand pit for them to play in. When they are older, bring their tricycles, bikes, or skates so they can wheel along beside you.

- **Playground:** Be a kid again and join your child on the playground. Swing, slide, crawl, climb, and laugh. But don't push the smaller kids out of the way, you bully.

- **Classes:** Sign up for a mom-and-tot exercise class. These classes are often offered through YMCA or churches and synagogues. If you're the only dad there, that's okay, too. Then people will just think you're a nice guy.

- **Musical Moves:** Find music that both you and your child enjoy and move to it. Be creative: toss a ball or march in time with the beat, move like animals, stop the music and "freeze," then start all over again. Again, these classes are offered through lots of community outlets. Or you can always just throw down a Fat Daddy Dance Party, where you crank the music and bust a move. Close the curtains first, though.

## Installing a New Offense with Your Partner

You won't ever find time for your partner—*you have to make it.* Many experts recommend that you make a weekly date night, get a baby-sitter, and get out of the house together. However, the reality is that this is easier said than done. So what can you do?

First, acknowledge to each other that life really has changed and that your relationship will play second string to the new baby in your home for at least the first year or two (or three or four). It's even normal for a dad to feel a little left out as his wife, now a new mother, gets swept up in the care and needs of the baby.

So when you're finally ready to play one-on-one coverage again with your mate, try these suggestions:

- **Strive for a real date night and arrange baby-sitting.** If cost is an issue—or if you'd just feel more comfortable leaving the baby with someone you know—look into starting a baby-sitting co-op. And remember, you don't have to have a full-fledged night on the town: The goal is simply to get some time alone with each other. So take a walk, grab a bite, go to the movies. Then make out.

- **Make a date night at home.** You don't need a sitter to really pay attention to each other. Once your baby has settled down for the night—or at least for a few hours—seize some together time. Resist collapsing on the couch and switching on the TV or doing more work. Sit together for some face-to-face time. Focusing on each other for as little as ten minutes can make a huge difference. All too often, new parents can forget even to make eye contact with each other. By simply carving out some moments just to be together you'll feel more connected and in touch. Also, make out.

- **Get creative.** You don't have to wait for the sun to go down to spend quality time with each other. For instance, commute together or have lunch together. It's surprising how animated conversation can become when you're meeting in the middle of the day and there's no baby or batch of chores to worry about. Plus, you can make out before the bill comes.

- **Send a love letter.** You don't have to pen Shakespearean prose to get your honey's heart pumping. You can say "I love you" with a quick e-mail, note, or voice mail. You virtual romantic devil, you.

- **Buy season tickets.** If you've already paid for seats at a concert, theater, or sporting event, you'll feel committed to going. To cut the cost, split the season tickets—and baby-sitting duties— with another couple that has a baby.

- **Treat weekends like weekends.** Pack the diaper bag, take out the stroller or a backpack, and enjoy a weekend activity as a family. Museums, malls, parks, outdoor events, and the like are all baby compatible.

- **Create some postwork rituals.** Try taking a walk together every evening with your baby. While your baby gets another walk or playtime, you two can really connect at day's end.

- **Plan your own rituals.** Start a weekly video and takeout dinner night. Once your baby settles into a predictable bedtime, life really changes (yet another great reason to work toward instituting a regular bedtime). Watching a video is an easy way to enjoy a little down time together. Or up time, depending on what you're watching.

- **Play games.** Games are a great way to connect, so dust off the chess set, a deck of cards, the Monopoly board, or whatever else you both enjoy playing.

- **Make time for yourself, too.** New parents really need alone-time before they can start giving to yet another person. Schedule this time first for your wife, then for yourself. It'll work out better that way.

## The Buffet and the Beast

Disney and doughnuts. Movies and Milkduds. It seems everywhere you turn companies are marketing sugar-laced sodas and greasy burgers to our kids. So much so, advertisers spend several hundred million dollars a year trying to influence our kids. If we as parents give in, then our kids lose. We have to be strong, be consistent, and help our kids make good food choices.

"I never see a child with better eating habits than his parents," says Keith Ayoob, associate professor of pediatrics at the Albert Einstein College of Medicine in New York. This is why parents have to not only be a good team in raising their children, but be "team captains" when it comes to making the hard calls on food

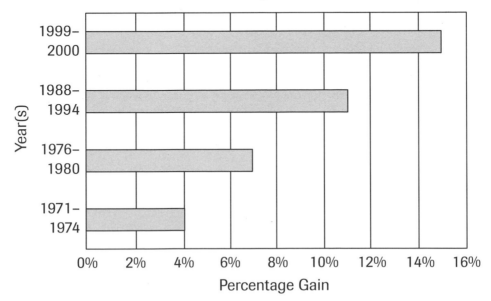

**Kids Packing on the Pounds**

and physical fitness. It's not only the extra pounds that can be unhealthy and lead to serious health problems like obesity and type 2 diabetes in our children, but chubby kids are often teased by their peers and develop low self-esteem.

To make it easy, just stick to these simple plays when showing the rookies (your kids) how to eat right.

- **Again, be a role model.** You eat five to seven servings of fruits and vegetables a day, and they'll follow.

- **Practice the rule of one.** Kids are going to eat junk. However, try to keep the bad foods down to one item per day (i.e., cookie, snow cone, ice cream).

- **Teach your child how to snack.** That's right. They don't need to give up snacks—they just need to eat snack foods that are nutritious, such as apple slices, orange wedges, carrot sticks, peanut butter on whole wheat crackers, and so on. Also, stock the fridge with grab snacks like grapes, oranges, and bananas.

- **Get them involved.** Kids are more likely to enjoy the food they personally prepare. Supervise them until they can do it by themselves.

- **Make changes gradually.** An example: Don't go from a cheese-burger straight to a tofu burger. Put a turkey burger in between.

- **Don't be too pushy.** Kids who are pushed to try new foods are less likely to try those foods again than children who decide to experiment for themselves. Parents who serve meals in a relaxed manner help minimize a child's negative emotions. So don't get too angry if they're not begging for brussels sprouts.

- **Apples and oranges.** An apple a day can definitely keep the doctor away. An extremely popular, practical, and tasty fruit, apples have medicinal properties to boot. They contain vitamins A and C, boron, and other goodies. They also have antibacterial and antiviral qualities. In addition, studies show that the smell of green apples reduces appetite. Certain alternative medicines use the scent of green apples to induce weight loss. As for oranges, they can help ward off nasty colds and flu because of their vitamin C levels. But did you know oranges also help prevent lung, stomach, pancreatic, colon, and breast cancer? It's true. On top of that, oranges also contain potassium and vitamin B, which help prevent strokes and heart disease. It is also believed that oranges raise fertility in men. And one or two oranges a day is all it takes.

- **Be like Bugs (Bunny).** Carrots are a potent medicinal food because of their beta-carotene content. Beta-carotene is linked with fighting cancer, strengthening the immune system and protecting arteries. One carrot a day can cut lung cancer risk in half, and the belief that carrots are good for the eyes is well founded—beta-carotene prevents eye diseases, such as cataracts. They also have a soothing effect on the stomach, reducing constipation and diarrhea. Plus, according to the *American Journal of Clinical Nutrition*, carrots cleanse the body by flushing out heavy metals from tissues. Sounds painful, don't it? But you'll actually never notice.

## For the Veterans (Most of You)

Even though we discussed food earlier in the second quarter, here are a couple other veteran tips that will help you practice what you preach to your teammates:

- **Eat clean.** If you can catch it, pluck it, or peel it, chances are your kids should eat it.

- **Stock up on produce.** Apples, berries, bananas, spinach, lettuce, dates, green beans, soybeans, and the like.

- **Get your grains.** Whole wheat breads and pastas, brown rice, flaxseed, whole grain cereals, oatmeal, grits, low-fat granola, and any type of bean (except refried).

- **Don't ignore the dairy.** Low- or nonfat milks, cheeses, and yogurts are all great sources of calcium and protein. Even low-fat ice cream is okay once in a while.

- **Drink up.** Water, real fruit juice, milk, green tea, and an occasional glass of red wine.

- **Don't troll.** If there are scraps left behind by your kids, toss them. An extra chicken nugget here, an extra slice of pizza there, and next thing you know you are hitting the next notch on your belt.

## Game Summary

Long before man discovered the treadmill and the Atkins diet, he lived in a time when vigorous physical activity was an intricate part of daily life. Inventions like cars, cell phones, and Palm Pilots have freed us from hard labor, but our bodies still need it. Combine that with the compelling research that "participating fathers" can enhance the nonverbal communication skills in infants and can help children develop empathy and self-control, it is our responsibility as fathers to lead by example by staying in shape with a proper diet and exercise regimen. Whether you are teaching your boy how to throw a ball or teaching him how to live a healthy life, it is our responsibility to set the bar.

Physical activity is not only important for our kids, but for all stages of our lives:

- In children, physical fitness aids in the development of coordination, strong bones and muscles, positive socialization, and positive self-image.

- With teens, exercise helps them feel independent, confident, and strong. It also reduces the onset of chronic diseases like osteoporosis and heart disease in adulthood.

- Dads and moms that are physically active maintain, and may even improve, their health, have a better sense of emotional well-being, and have more control over their weight.

- With older folks, physical activity helps to keep bones and muscles, including the heart, strong. It also aids digestion, fights depression, and improves alertness.

"When you exercise, you feel your heart rate go up, you get anxious and jittery, and the brain's recognition has a psychological experience," says Jay Smith, Ph.D., a sports medicine physiatrist at the Mayo Clinic in Rochester, Minnesota. That's actually a good thing, even if it doesn't sound like it. Dr. Smith's point is that exercise makes our brains work faster and our bodies work better. And with a fit body, clear mind, and a strong commitment to family, we Fat Daddies will have the fundamentals that can lead our team to victory!

## PLAYBOOK NOTES: Family—The Fundamentals

1. Be a role model. Studies indicate that there's a direct relationship between how active children become as adults and the level of physical activity they saw in their parents while growing up. (What a strong enticement for you to get active!)

2. Get off the couch. Take a break from TV by planning one family physical activity outing a week. Let your child help pick the activity and location. Check out classes you can take together, such as karate.

3. As parents, you and your partner are team captains. So call the right plays when it comes to teaching healthy habits to your kids.

4. Take time to install a new offense with your partner. Be smart. Beauty fades, but dumb is forever.

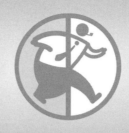

# How the Game Is Won

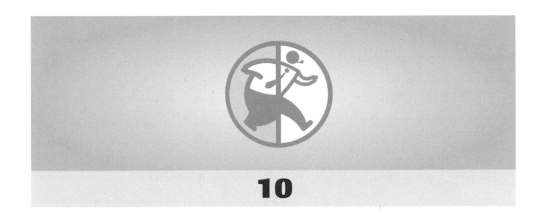

**10**

# Implementing the Game Plan

"Setting a goal is not the main thing. It is deciding how you will
go about achieving it and staying with that plan."

—TOM LANDRY, coaching legend of the Dallas Cowboys

his is it. Game time. You know the plays already. We've practiced them over the past many pages. And you know by now
that there is no magic here. No point systems, no cabbage soup—
unless you like cabbage soup, you freak. No, the Fat Daddy game
plan is all about the basics—Family, Food, Fitness. You remember
what we've practiced, right? Four to six meals a day. Exercise six
days a week, one hour per day. Involve the whole family in fitness.
Get healthy for yourself, so your wife and kids will get and stay
healthy, too. That all sounds familiar, doesn't it? It better. Because
we're about to hit the field and you need to execute to win. So, just
to be sure, let's review the basics one more time.

## Key Plays

### Family—The Fundamentals

- **Lead by example.** As a father, it is your job to set the right example for the wife and children and to help them find the time and resources to get in shape *with* you.

- **Make it fun.** The best way to stay in shape is to vary your workout.

- **Just do it—together.** It's a team game.


### Fitness—The Framework

- **A time and a place.** The gym, at home, at the office, in a car—there are many places you can sneak in exercise.

- **Four quarters.** Stretching, cardio, weights, and yoga. You have to find a way to squeeze them all in every week.


### Food—The Foundation

- **Frequent the training table.** What, how much, and how often? Eat four to six small, somewhat healthy meals a day.

- **Be handy.** Never eat more than your open hand at one sitting. Or, more precisely, never eat more than the *volume* of your open hand.

- **You are what you eat.** If you can catch it, pick it, or pluck it you're probably okay.


## Automatic Plays

Okay, so that's the big picture. You know what the team concept is all about. But you also need to know the core plays, the concepts you can fall back on in any situation when the game is on the line. These ten plays are the grease in the Fat Daddy wheels, the fuel in the Fat Daddy rocket, the cabbage in the Fat Daddy soup—er, well, make that the meat in the Fat Daddy sandwich. Yeah, that's what they are. Do them all, do them well, and, again, you'll win.

1. **Work it.** Try to get some exercise in every day—six minutes to sixty minutes, something is better than nothing. When parking your car, try parking a little farther away. Also, try taking the stairs at work.

2. **Size it up.** If you go to a restaurant and your portions are too large, cut them in half.

3. **Go slow and steady.** Always try to eat slowly. It takes about twenty minutes for the signal indicating that you're full to go from your stomach to your brain. By slowing your pace, you'll avoid overeating. Try chewing each bite at least ten times.

4. **Eat more often.** Aside from portion control, the frequency of your meals is also important. Simply put: more meals on smaller plates. Just remember to eat five small meals a day instead of three big ones.

5. **Drink up.** Fill your tank with at least eight glasses of water a day.

6. **Cut back on the comfort.** Sweets, alcohol, bread, pasta. Lot's of empty calories and carbs are not worth the taste.

7. **Don't eat after 8:00 P.M.** No matter what, 7:59 P.M. and not a minute later. What your body can't process, it stores as fat.

8. **Up and at 'em.** When at work, get up every hour or so and walk around. Even five minutes is enough to get the blood flowing.

9. **Play with the team.** Just getting out and playing with your kids will help you burn more calories.

10. **Get some shut-eye.** Nothing robs good progress like lack of sleep. No matter when you go to bed—early or late—try to get at least eight hours a night.

## Trick Plays

The halfback pass, the end around, the flea flicker, the Statue of Liberty, the Foro Romani, and, well, you get the idea. Except maybe for the last one, they're all trick plays. The things you'll go to when the defense is getting tough and seems to be in your path at every turn. When that happens, you throw these plays at your opponents— whether those opponents are your kids at homework time, your wife at nagging hour (aka sunup to sundown), or yourself when you're feeling slothy. The trick plays are:

- **Do yoga.** There has been a great deal of research that yoga can lower cholesterol, increase strength and flexibility. If you have to pick one type of exercise, this should be it.

- **Exercise as a family.** Showing your kids that exercise can be fun will become one of the most impressionable acts that will promote their fitness habits in years to come. Better that they do bench presses than Burger King.

- **Be in tune with your spouse.** If you and your spouse are happy, everybody is happy. Think of your marriage as the hub, and everything else in life is the spokes. If the hub is unstable, all of the spokes collapse. So get yourself a screwdriver and tighten things up, if you know what I mean.

## Blind Side

Look out. BLITZ! The sad truth is that the munchkins often arrive with the speed of Deion Sanders and the ferocity of Dick

Butkus. You're looking downfield one second and the next you're looking down at your broken face mask. Kids blindside you and your spouse. And, sadly, 70 percent of couples that have kids become less satisfied with their marriage after the children are born. Stress, lack of sleep, and the added responsibilities of parenting are clearly to blame and not the kids themselves. But there are several ways to protect that blind side and keep your relationship from souring:

- **Get involved.** Help your wife with the traditional "mom-type" duties. Changing the diapers, driving the car pool, cleaning the house, and dressing the kids all help ease the stress around the house.

- **Listen up.** Pay attention to your partner's "minor" bids for attention and affection. A simple kiss, touch of a shoulder, or listening to what happened at work today will pay huge dividends!

- **Rumble right.** Research has shown that couples who use a collaborative style of arguing—expressing their opinions and trying to reach a mutually acceptable conclusion instead of trying to "win" an argument—have a much happier and more trusting relationship.

- **Stay pals.** Studies have shown the secret to any long-term relationship is friendship. So go play catch or something, for crying out loud.

- **Concede defeat.** It is important to recognize that there will be hard times. Successful couples don't live in Disneyland, they don't even live in Euro Disneyland. Instead, couples that stick it out accept that some days together will simply flat-out suck. They accept that and adapt accordingly.

■ **Get it on.** You do it. You love to do it. I just did it and I'm ready to do it again. Yes, like Mr. Brooks said, it's good to be the king. But, yeah, it can be hard to find the time, sometimes even the motivation, to "do it" once you're married with children. Your partner is the same. You're the same. But, still, you know you want it. So follow the researchers' advice, and accept that it is the responsibility of *both* partners to be a little creative from time to time in the bedroom. Fat Daddy suggests trying a game of "Star Quarterback meets Head Cheerleader."

## Man-to-Man Coverage

A man's gotta do what a man's gotta do. And sometimes he's gotta do that on his own. Yes, it's your blubber, bub. You have to be responsible for trimming it. Here's a review on how to do that without upsetting your family:

■ **Make time for exercise.** Earlier in the morning or later in the evening—it doesn't matter. Just get at least one hour of exercise at least six days a week.

■ **Do it together.** Couples that work out together stay together.

■ **Eat dinner early.** If you eat after 8:00 P.M., you will gain weight. Plus, having a consistent time for dinner together is great for communicating and bonding.

## Coffin Corner

Okay, boys, no lectures here. Just the facts. Guys are harder on their bodies than women. We live harder and die faster. But it doesn't have to be that way. Try these simple tips, and you'll stick around to spoil your grandkids:

- **Control your circumference.** Obesity kills over 300,000 people per year.

- **Don't smoke.** Smoking kills over 400,000 people per year.

- **Wear sunscreen.** SPF every day, or have your skin removed piece by piece by your dermatologist in a few years.

- **Take a baby aspirin every day.** Will help reduce the risk of strokes, heart attacks, and other clotting type problems.

- **Eat right.** That means more protein, good fats, and fewer carbs.

- **Wear a raincoat.** AIDS can kill you.

- **Work out regularly.** Got the point yet?

- **Get tested—The Fat Daddy Fab Five:**

  1. **Colon cancer:** Have a colonoscopy every five years after age forty.

  2. **Heart disease:** Check cholesterol and blood pressure twice a year.

  3. **Glaucoma:** Test vision every year.

  4. **Testicular cancer:** Get a testicular exam twice a year.

  5. **Skin cancer:** Have an annual exam from a dermatologist.

- **Relax.** Find a quiet place, and sit quiet for at least ten minutes. Try it every day. You'll be amazed how you feel after!

## Touchdown

I hope you enjoyed Fat Daddy. I tried to make it an easy read that outlined a realistic eating plan, offered a simple exercise regimen, and provided a few tips on how to balance family and work. The *Keys to the Game* are easy to under-stand, easy to follow, easy to remember, and will serve as a playbook to help busy dads cinch in that belt a couple notches without a great deal of diet or workout sorcery.

> "Too many men equate husbandhood with fatherhood, much to the detriment of their kids. Being a father is so much more."
>
> – MARSHA A. KANHOFF, LMSW-ACP, LMFT

Regardless what kind of Fat Daddy you are, the fact that you are a daddy means you're a role model for your family. You have to lead by example, have to become a true partner in tune with your wife, have to find time to work out, have to eat the right foods, and have to be an involved father. You have to do all of that every day on every down. Not because I told you so but because you want to. You want to win. And you can.

Good luck dad, I'm pulling for you.

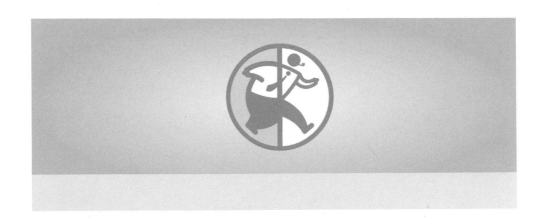

# Resources

Although there are aisles and aisles of health and wellness books at your local bookstore, most Fat Daddies do not have the time to do the legwork. Hence, here are a group of websites that I have found to be very informative and useful.

| MEN'S FITNESS | |
|---|---|
| AskMen.com | www.askmen.com |
| Fat Daddy | www.fatdaddy.com |
| Fitness Online | www.fitnessonline.com |
| Men's Fitness | www.mensfitness.com |
| Men's Health | www.menshealth.com |
| The Men's Center | www.themenscenter.com |

## FATHERHOOD

| | |
|---|---|
| Dads and Pregnancy | www.thelaboroflove.com/forum/doug/1.html |
| Fatherville | www.fatherville.com |
| National Fatherhood Initiative | www.fatherhood.org |
| NCF (National Center for Fathering) | www.fathers.com |
| U.S. Department of Health and Human Services—Fathers | www.fatherhood.hhs.gov |

## HEALTH AND WELLNESS

| | |
|---|---|
| Ask-a-Doctor | www.askadoctor.com |
| Dr. Weil | www.drweil.com |
| Intellihealth | www.intellihealth.com |
| MedScape | www.medscape.com |
| Natural Health | www.naturalhealthmag.com |
| Net Live MD | www.netlivemd.com |
| On Health Network Co. | www.onhealth.com |
| The Cooper Center | www.cooperaerobics.com |
| The Mayo Clinic | www.mayoclinic.com |
| ThriveOnline | www.thriveonline.com |
| WebMD | www.webmd.com |

## ONLINE DIETS AND EXERCISE PROGRAMS

| | |
|---|---|
| Cyber Diet | www.bodyfatguide.com |
| eDiets | www.ediets.com |
| eNutrition | www.enutrition.com |
| Jenny Craig | www.jennycraig.com |
| Nutrio | www.nutrio.com |
| Real Age | www.realage.com |
| Shape Up! | www.shapeup.org |
| Slim-Fast | www.slim-fast.com |
| The Zone Diet | www.enterthezone.com |
| Weight Watchers | www.weightwatchers.com |

## ASSOCIATIONS AND REFERENCE

| | |
|---|---|
| American Cancer Society | www.cancer.org |
| American Diabetes Association | www.diabetes.org |
| American Heart Association | www.americanheart.org |
| American Medical Association | www.ama-assn.org |
| American Psychological Association | www.apa.org |
| Center for Nutrition and Policy Promotion | www.usda.gov |

*(Continued)*

## ASSOCIATIONS AND REFERENCE (Continued)

| | |
|---|---|
| Food and Nutrition Information Center | www.nal.usda.gov |
| National Cancer Institute | www.cancer.gov |
| President's Counsel on Physical Fitness | http://fitness.gov |
| Reuter's Health Information Services | www.reutershealth.com |
| The American Society for Clinical Nutrition | www.faseb.org |
| The American Society for Nutritional Sciences | www.asns.org |
| The Center for Disease Control | www.cdc.gov |

## CHILDREN AND FAMILY

| | |
|---|---|
| American Academy of Child and Adolescent Psychiatry | www.aacap.org |
| American Council on Exercise | www.acefitness.org |
| Cool Nurse | www.coolnurse.com |
| Kids Health | www.kidshealth.com |
| Pediatric Planet | www.pediatricplanet.com |
| YMCA | www.ymca.org |

| GUY STUFF | |
|---|---|
| Brooks Brothers (clothes) | www.brooksbrothers.com |
| Brookstone (cool stuff) | www.brookstone.com |
| Car and Driver (cars) | www.caranddriver.com |
| Grooms Online (gifts) | www.groomsonline.com |
| Guyville (gifts and such) | www.weddingstand.com |
| Hammacher (cool stuff) | www.hammacher.com |
| Kiehls (grooming products) | www.keihls.com |
| Maxim (content) | www.maxim.com |
| Moma (cool stuff) | www.momastore.com |
| Moss (cool furniture stuff) | www.mossonline.com |
| Movie Quotes | www.moviequotes.com |
| Nike | www.nike.com |
| Online Sports Collectibles (sports gifts) | www.onlinesports.com |
| Pink (clothing) | www.thomaspink.com |
| Rand McNally (maps and stuff) | www.randmcnally.com |
| Room & Board (cool furniture stuff) | www.roomandboard.com |
| Stuff (content) | www.stuffmagazine.com |

*(Continued)*

## GUY STUFF (Continued)

| | |
|---|---|
| The Art of Shaving (grooming products) | www.theartofshaving.com |
| The Divorce Source (divorce) | www.divorcesource.com |
| The Knot (wedding gifts) | www.theknot.com |
| The Sharper Image (cool stuff) | www.sharperimage.com |
| The Wedding Channel (gift registry) | www.weddingchannel.com |
| Weather (weather reports and the like) | www.weather.com |
| Wine.com (wine) | www.wine.com |
| Zipper (cools stuff) | www.zippergifts.com |

## BABY/FAMILY STUFF

| | |
|---|---|
| A Baby (fancy baby stuff) | www.ababy.com |
| Baby Gap (clothes) | www.babygap.com |
| eStyle/Baby Style (clothes) | www.babystyle.com |
| Fit Pregnancy | www.fitpregnancy.com |
| Gymboree (clothes) | www.gymboree.com |
| Old Navy (clothes) | www.oldnavy.com |

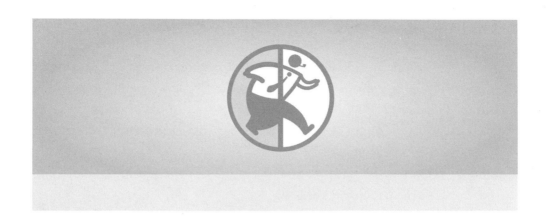

# References

Acheson, K., Y. Schultz, T. Bessard, et al. (1984). Nutritional influences on lipogenesis and thermogenesis after a carbohydrate meal. *American Journal of Physiology* 246(1): E62-70.

Belko, A. (1987) Vitamins and exercise: an update. *Medicine and Science in Sports and Exercise* 19: S191-S196.

Connelly, Scott A., and Carol Colman (2001). *Body Rx*. New York: Putnam's.

Cooper, K. (1982). *The Aerobics Program for Total Well Being: Exercise, Diet, Emotional Balance*. New York: M. Evans.

Costill, D., G. Dalsky, and W. Fink (1978). Effects of caffeine ingestion on metabolism and exercise performance. *Medicine in Science in Sports and Exercise* 10(3): 155–158.

Editors of Men's Health Books (1999). *The Complete Guide to Men's Health*: *The Definitive, Illustrated Guide to Healthy Living, Exercise, and Sex*. Emmaus, Pa.: Rodale Press, pp. 4, 18, 49, 132.

Griffith, H. Winter, Dan Levinson, and Gail Harrison (1988). *Complete Guide to Vitamins, Minerals, and Supplements*. Tuscon, Ariz.: Fisher Books.

Hakkien, K. (1989). Neuromuscular and hormonal adaptations during strength and power training: a review. *Journal of Sports Medicine and Physical Fitness* 29(11): 9–26.

Is it necessary to cut back on salt after all? (1988). *Tufts University Diet and Nutritional News Letter* 6, no. 6.

Ivy, J. (1988). Muscle glycogen synthesis after exercise: effect of time of carbohydrate ingestion. *Journal of Applied Physiology* 64: 1480-1485.

Johnson, Timothy (2002). *Dr. Timothy Johnson's On Call Guide to Men's Health: Authoritative Answers to Your Most Important Questions.* New York: Hyperion, pp. 22–25, 36–39.

Kirshman, J. D., and Lavon J. Dunne (1984). *The Nutrition Almanac,* 2nd ed. New York: McGraw-Hill.

Kleiner, S. M. (1996). In high spirits? Alcohol and your health. *The Physician and Sports Medicine* 24(9).

Lehu, P., and T. Iknoian (2000). *Mind-Body Fitness for Dummies.* Indianapolis: IDG Books.

Leiber, C. S. (1995). The nutritional effects of alcohol. In *Total Nutrition: The Only Guide You'll Ever Need.* New York: St. Martin's Press, 348–358.

Lombardo, J. A. (1986). Stimulants and athletic performance: cocaine and nicotine. *The Physician and Sports Medicine* 14(12): 85–89.

Lukashi, H. C. (1987) Methods of assessment of the human body composition. *American Journal of Clinical Nutrition* 46, 537.

Mindell, E. (1985). *Earl Mindell's Vitamin Bible for the 21st Century,* rev. ed. New York: Warner.

National Institutes of Health (1998). Clinical guidelines on the identification, evaluation, and treatment of overweight and obesity in adults. Bethesda, Md.: Department of Health and Human Services, National Institutes of Health, National Heart, Lung, and Blood Institute.

National Research Council (1998). *Diet and Health: Implications for Reducing Chronic Disease Risk.* Washington, DC: National Academy Press, 1989.

Nelson, K. (1953). *The Daddy Guide: Real-Life Advice and Tips from over 250 Dads and Other Experts.* Lincolnwood, Ill.: Contemporary Books.

Paris, B. (1996). *Natural Fitness.* New York: Warner Books.

Robbins, Anthony (1986). *Unlimited Power: The New Science of Personal Achievement.* New York: Simon & Schuster.

Sherman, W., D. Costill, W. Fink, and J. Miller (1981). Effect of exercise-diet manipulation on muscle glycogen and its subsequent utilization during performance. *International Journal of Sports Medicine* 2, 114–118.

Stewart, M., J. McDonald, A. Levy, et al. (1985). Vitamin/mineral supplement use. *Journal of the American Dietetic Association* 85(12): 1585–1590.

Stunkard A. J., and T. A. Wadden, editors (1993). *Obesity: Theory and Therapy,* 2nd ed. New York: Raven Press.

University of Virginia (YEAR). Cycling fat. *Journal of Sports Science* 13(4): 204–207.

Williams, M. (1984) Vitamin and mineral supplements to athletes: do they help? *Clinics in Sports Medicine* 3(3): 623–637.

Wilmore, J. H., and D. L. Costill (1994). *Physiology of Sport and Exercise.* Champaign, Ill.: Human Kinetics.

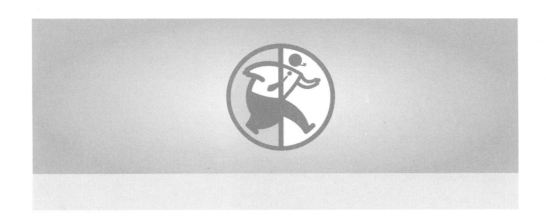

# Index

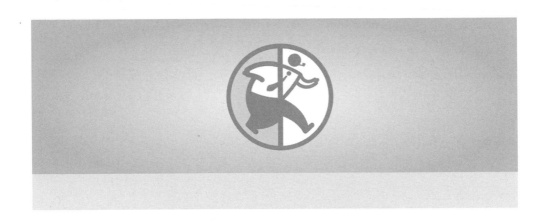

# About the Author

A former Fat Daddy, **Lawrence Schwartz** is president of Skywire Software, an exercise enthusiast, a syndicated columnist of "Ask Fat Daddy," a recipient of the 2003 Father of the Year Award, and a dad who lives for his kids, Cole and Cameron.